GOOD VIBRATIONS

Good Vibrations

Overcoming
S*pasmodic* **D***ysphonia*

Ken McDonald B.D., Th.M.

First Edition

Copyright ©2017 Ken McDonald
All Rights Reserved

ISBN 978-1-942769-06-4

Printed in the United States of America

All Rights Reserved. No part of this publication may be reproduced, stored in a retrieval system, or transmitted in any form by any means, electronic, mechanical, photocopy, recording or otherwise, without the prior written permission of the publisher, except for brief quotations in critical reviews or articles.

Cover Design: Ken and Terri Lee McDonald
Cover Photo: Shutterstock.com

Acknowledgements

I would like to say thank you to Bill Rooks and Jean Clark for their help in editing, as well as a great thank you to my dear wife, Terri, for her help and constant encouragement and faithfulness through the very difficult years when my voice was gone.

Unfortunate!

It is unfortunate to have to write the following.

I have previously written this book under a different title. I wrote it originally as an instructional book of how to perform these exercises to restore your voice. Along with that I mentioned the name of my voice instructor who greatly helped me over those years, but unfortunately after the book was published, I was contacted by their office with the threat of lawsuit for writing the book. This took me by surprise as I was only trying to help people who had lost their voice as well as mentioning who had helped me.

I have had to rewrite this book in a first person testimony as well as removing all references to who it was that instructed me in these exercises. In some spots the wording may seem awkward. This is why.

Disclaimer

I am not a doctor, a speech therapist, or medical provider of any kind. I am a man who, after being diagnosed at the University of Pittsburgh Medical Center by Dr. Clark Rosen with Abductor Spasmodic Dysphonia, used this system of vocal training and exercises to rehabilitate my voice. This book is about what I went through and is not intended for diagnostic use, treatment or to determine anything medically about you or your voice. If your voice is not working the way it should, then you need to be examined by a proper medical doctor.

I do not recommend alternative metaphysical medicine doctors whatsoever, and I have written a book titled *Defiled*, which explains my position on that matter.

Other Books
By
Ken McDonald B.D., Th.M.,

Here Comes The Bride
A Critique of the Baptist Bride Heresy

Pursuit
One Man's Quest to Find
God's Perfect Will for His Life

Defiled
The Spiritual Dangers
of Alternative Medicine

Jesus, Talk To Me
Have you ever wanted to get God's attention?
(Sermon in a Book Series, Vol. 1)

Dealing With Bad In-Laws
A Bible Study on Jacob and Laban
(Sermon in a Book Series, Vol. 2)

Even As God
Healing Relationships Biblically
(Sermon in a Book Series, Vol. 3)

Table of Contents

Chapter	Page
Preface	13
Introduction	15
1. My Story	19
2. Some Things You Should Know	33
3. The Three Modalities	41
4. Practical Tips For Voice	53
5. What Are You Doing?	57
6. My First Exercise & Daily Workout	77
7. 2nd Workout - Third or Forth Week	83
8. 3rd Workout - Third Month	85
9. 4th Workout - Six Months	95
10. For The Very Weak Voice	101
11. 5th Workout - One Year	109
12. Two Year Mark	115
13. Extra Exercises	127
14 The Exercises Illustrated	133
15. A Glimpse of the Path	147

Table of Contents

Chapter	Page
16. Origin of the Smolover Method	191
17. The Most Important Step	197
18. Bibliography	213

Preface

Many people have heard of my experience by word of mouth. From time to time, I receive requests from folks who have voice troubles and who want to have their voices restored. So I send them exercises and additional information based on what I did personally to overcome Spasmodic Dysphonia (SD). My heart goes out to these folks because I know what it's like to be without a voice.

As the requests for help grew in number, I prayed and realized that the need for this information is widespread enough to warrant writing this book. Whether it merely speaks to your heart or provides real and lasting help for your own broken voice, my desire is to let you know that you are not alone and that there is help to be had.

The past few years of having my voice back have been wonderful, but as I began to work on the book I was reminded of the frustration, discouragement and general upheaval that occurs when the voice is absent. I remembered the years in my own life when I would sit alone in my bedroom not wanting to see or attempt to talk to anyone. Yes, I know what it feels like not having a voice.

This book may only be a layman's attempt at explaining the Smolover method, but this layman has "walked this road." I will attempt to describe my road to recovery using this method.

I am not the only person who has suffered from SD and recovered. There are others who have been diagnosed with either Abductor type SD or Adductor type SD, who are now talking again because of this method of vocal exercise. Lord willing, you can find similar success.

Introduction

Whether this small book will be received with approval or disdain I do not know. (Perhaps it will be both depending on the realm in which it is distributed.) What I do know is that I was once unable to talk, and that two extremely proficient and recognized doctors diagnosed me with SD. Their names are Dr. Clark Rosen and Dr. Jackie Gartner-Schmidt, of the University of Pittsburgh Medical Center. Both of these doctors are among the best in their respective fields.

I also know that, today, I can speak and talk freely. The frustration, fear, seclusion and discouragement from not having a voice are gone. I am back at work, which involves lively public speaking, and my voice is holding up very well. I have gone from not being able to talk on the

Good Vibrations

phone, in a crowd, or even at home, to public speaking, at times without a PA system for help. I am also singing in public as well, which is something I never even considered when my voice was gone.

I know that the Smolover method has worked for me, and others who have been guided through the workouts by a few other Vocal Behavior Training instructors. This is my story and testimony and I am confident that if you have Spasmodic Dysphonia there is a good possibility that you can also talk once again through performing these exercises that make up the Smolover Method.

Though fifty years in the making, as you will see, the theory behind the method is simple and, in my view, very logical.

As mentioned in the opening disclaimer, I am not a doctor. I am merely telling my personal story and what I learned in the process; what has worked for me. For three years, I was immersed into this therapy by attending one-hour sessions up to three times a week. For two years after that I was in sessions when I was able to attend. I still

> "...most professionals believe that success in voice therapy is defined as a return to a functional level of voicing..."[1]
>
> Dr. Jackie Gartner-Schmidt

Introduction

to this day work my voice, though not as often as I should. I have gone from not being able to talk to returning to public speaking as well as to singing.

Do I still have SD? Yes! But I am able to function as a result of these exercises, and that is a great blessing!

If you are reading this and are suffering from SD it is likely that you can get your voice back, not by gimmicks or "Band-Aids." These exercises work. However, I will tell you quite plainly: it is going to take a lot of effort on your part. They are very challenging to perform and it takes time, but I know it works because I have done it. And if I can do it, so can you.

1

My Story

Perhaps you are not really all that interested in reading my story. You want to know how to get your voice back. I understand! You can skip this for now and move on, but I would recommend reading my testimony so you know what I have been through and will know I understand where you are at.

I understand the frustration, fear, seclusion and discouragement that come from not being able to speak. I know what it is like, and now that I have my voice back it is amazing how I had to stop and think of what it was like to not have a voice. Yes, my voice is that much better. Most of the time I do not, and am not, aware that my voice was bad.

Good Vibrations

It had been a long trip; thirty-two hours from the time I left Buffalo, New York, until I arrived at the missionary's front door step in Lipa City, Philippines. I was exhausted and, on top of that, the time change was almost opposite of what I was used to.

I rested as best I could for a few hours, and then the meeting started. It was a preaching meeting in a barangay, which is a small village, in the hills just south of Lipa City. The second evening of the meeting my voice gave out. I was one of the main speakers and I had no voice! What was I going to do?

That night they put together a makeshift public address system, and I literally kept my lips on the microphone and whispered a sermon into it. That was the first time my voice ever gave out, and it was never the same after that.

I was in my early forties and had been doing meetings constantly for about four years prior to my voice giving out. At the time I didn't think all that much about it, but little did I know it was evidence that something was very wrong with my voice. As a driver that has no idea the bridge that is just around the next bend has been washed out, I too had no idea that in the ensuing years my voice would grow weaker and weaker and then collapse.

When I first started traveling and speaking in churches across America, I thought nothing of the

My Story

weakness of my voice. My family and I would arrive back home in the Sierra Nevada Mountains of Central California, and we would rest from the grueling rigors of life on the road. After a week of rest at home my voice would come back good as new.

The next year it would take two weeks for my voice to fully recover. I just figured I was a little more tired than the previous year, but it came back so all was good. The third year of being out on the road and speaking we came home and rested. My voice came back, but not all the way. It wasn't like it was good as new, but I thought little of it, though I did notice it. Then I took that trip to the Philippines. When you are in the middle of it all, you don't see what is happening.

At many of my speaking engagements I play guitar and sing. During those years my two children were with my wife, Terri, and I on the road and we would sing as a family. As time went by I was not able to sing as much because my voice could not reach the notes. It just kept getting worse and worse.

I began to ask other Pastors what they did for their voices. I wondered if they had some sort of remedy. Often though people would come up to me and offer cough drops because it sounded like I had a cold. Other "remedies" ranged from tea and honey; room temperature tea that is, but it didn't help. One Pastor told me to try Sen-Sen,

Good Vibrations

which is an old time candy consisting of licorice flavored breath bits. This helped a little for a short time and then ceased to help. I tried Aloe vera juice diluted in water, but that was no help. The absolute worst so-called remedy of them all was the North Carolina preachers' suggestion to drink the juice of a fresh lemon that had been mixed with Cayenne pepper. Oh, that was horrible! It did not help either. The one other "remedy" that I did not try was straight moonshine or whiskey. All such home remedies do one of two things. They either soothe your vocal cords or they clean the vocal cords. But because the problem with my vocal cords was neither dirty cords nor irritated cords, none of these "remedies" worked for me.

The best help I found was to drink a large amount (at least sixty-four ounces) of water two hours before stepping into the pulpit. This meant, though, that I had to have been to the rest room just prior to stepping into the pulpit. Oh, my! There were some close calls by the time I finished my sermon. Some of the sermons had to be cut short out of necessity, though I tried not to do that.

Nevertheless, my voice proceeded to grow worse. I began to avoid crowds, which is not a good thing for a preacher. I would let the pastor know that I would enter the church just before stepping into the pulpit, and that I would leave immediately

My Story

when I was finished preaching. I was unable to talk to anyone if I had to compete with surrounding noise, so I removed myself from those situations.

It became so frustrating if I tried to speak. I would try to stay relaxed and speak. Because they couldn't hear me they would ask, "What was that?" So I would try to raise my voice so they could hear me and nothing would come out.

In these situations, I relied on my wife. She generally knew what I was trying to say and would do my talking for me. Sometimes I resorted to writing things down on paper in order to communicate.

At one point a church in Los Angeles graciously paid for me to see an ENT (ear, nose and throat doctor) there, so I went. He scoped me, and oh, isn't that a joy! The last time he scoped me the scope was frayed on the camera end and scraped the inside of my nasal passage all the way in. I just wondered what particles of the last patient were imbedded within the frayed end.

Well, anyway, his diagnosis was Pharyngitis, and his prescription was that I needed to not talk for three months. Now I had been around hospitals in a previous job and I knew that "-itis" meant irritated. Pharynx was my pharynx, that's pretty plain. So his diagnosis was that my pharynx was irritated. Whoopee!

I retired back to a church in Yuma, Arizona, and

stayed there for four months with orders to only whisper. My vocal cords were not to make sound. I gave it four months instead of three just to make sure all was well.

When the four months were up, I gathered my family, and we set out for my next meeting. The first night of the meeting I began to speak and, five minutes into my sermon, I knew my voice had not improved one bit. It was as poor in quality as the day before I started my four months of silence. I was in the middle of my sermon, but I almost had a split personality, for I was delivering my sermon, but fear had gripped my mind as I wondered what was going to happen? Was I going to lose my voice? How would I support my family? What was I going to do? I had no answers. The only thing I could do was press on, and so I did.

My voice continued to decline to a state of weakness and hoarseness that moved me to silence as much as possible. The condition even created in me a frustrated anger whenever I had to talk. I was resigned to live a secluded life. It would be a life where verbal communication would be kept to the utmost minimum.

My wife, Terri, encouraged me to go to a specialist to find out what the problem was with my voice. I prayed about it and after much research, I decided to go to the University of Pittsburgh Medical Center where Dr. Clark Rosen was practicing. I had no idea how I was going to pay for the appointment, but the need was such that I stepped out by faith. After the first day of testing, a church in Tennessee called and told me they had taken up an offering for the testing. It was more than enough to cover the expense. That was a great comfort! Thank you Lord!

After two days of extensive testing I was diagnosed with Abductor type Spasmodic Dysphonia, with some Adductor Dysphonia as well. Though both types seem opposites there are those rare cases where both types are present. The doctors told me that speech therapy would not help, or help very little, and that the recommended treatment would be Botox injections.

The explanation (as I understood it) was that my nerves were over-stimulating the muscles and causing them to pull the vocal cords apart. Botox would deaden the nerve ends, thus enabling the muscles to relax and bring the vocal cords together so that they would vibrate normally to make sound. As the nerves would grow new ends, the problem with my voice would return. My voice would grow breathy again, and they would need to inject Botox again to deaden the nerve ends. The process would cycle through over and over for the rest of my life.

I declined the treatment. What was I going to do? I didn't know, but I would only do Botox as my last resort.

Good Vibrations

    Continuing on the best I could, I grew more and more reclusive, frustrated and concerned about my future as a preacher. I was waiting for the day when I would finish a sermon, leave the pulpit and have someone walk up to me after a sermon and say, "I can't understand what you are saying." My public speaking became a 45-minute battle and struggle just to make sound. I felt like a barking dog when I spoke. In effect, I was slamming my vocal cords together while pushing air through my throat in order to get any sound to come out. After a speaking service I was exhausted, frustrated, and discouraged. I didn't want to talk to or see anyone. I couldn't talk on the phone, nor could I even talk to anyone in person.

    Finally, at one Sunday meeting not much different than any other, I attempted to preach a sermon in a church. After the service a man came up to me and asked, "What is wrong with your voice?" I told him that I had been diagnosed with SD. Though he did not have SD, he had gone to a voice teacher for voice help and told me about her. At this point I was very closed minded to any supposed helps. But when he told me that she had helped men who worked on the floor of the New York Stock Exchange I perked up my ears. Men who work on the floor of the NYSE yell often and hard. I thought to myself, if she can help them, then maybe she could help me.

My Story

The man contacted her on my behalf and told her that I would be calling to make an appointment soon. When I made the call, what impressed me most was her confidence that she could help me, and that I would be fine. This astounded me, as no one else had ever been that confident. One other thing that amazed me was that, in less than two minutes of talking to her on the phone, she told me that I had SD without my having revealed the Pittsburg doctors' diagnosis.

My first two lessons with her went something like this: She had me lightly hum outward as she played a note on her piano. This, she followed by the next higher note and so on, until she had worked with me for an hour. After those first two sessions, my voice was much better, and I was amazed.

I departed for my next series of meetings and was much excited about the progress with my voice. It was working as it did four to five years earlier. I was ecstatic! The progress, however, was short lived and after a week my voice continued to decline. (This is not uncommon for people who try the exercises but the improvement does not last, which was what happened to me.)

Then in May of 2005, that which I had feared and was waiting for, finally came to pass. A lady came up to me after the Sunday morning service and said, "Brother McDonald, I can't understand you." It's no wonder for I myself felt like a

Good Vibrations

barking dog just to get sound to come out. But after she said this I knew I was done.

Upon canceling all of my upcoming commitments for three months out, in June of 2005, I started voice rehab. Twice each week, I went to her for one-hour sessions. To me, it was an hour of near torture. Calmly, she would tell me to hum as she played a note. I would hum and then choke and cough. At times the choking was so hard I would see stars and nearly pass out. Beads of sweat would build up on my forehead, and my shirt would be wet by the end of each session.

The worst was when she started me on the intoning, or humming inward. For certain notes I would lean slightly forward, brace myself, empty my lungs, and with all the strength I could find I would hum inward when she played the note. I would cough, choke, and sigh over and over, for each note, as she proceeded to "wake up my ligament." My wife, Terri, would drive the hour-long commute home, and then I would work my voice there on my own.

On my way to voice lessons I could not even ask for a toll receipt, so I would look to my wife, and she would speak up from the passenger side and ask, "May we get a receipt, please?" Sometimes tears would come to my eyes as I walked into my teacher's office due to the fear that I would never get my voice back.

My Story

Three months passed, and then three more. During those first three months I was warned that my voice might get worse before it got better, and so it did. Fear gripped my mind as I began to think the exercises were going to ruin my voice, or make it even worse, but I had nowhere else to go. With determination I continued working my voice.

After six months there was a slight improvement that excited me greatly. New exercises were added, and I would go home and work my voice each day. After a year I asked my teacher if I could get out and preach. My voice was better, though not perfect, and I was chomping at the bit to get back to preaching. She would not tell me yes or no, but said it was my decision to make. I decided to give it a try.

We embarked on a preaching trip to Minnesota, and then on to Arizona. After two months out, my voice collapsed while in Arizona. My heart was broken, but I knew what I had to do. I cancelled the rest of my meetings and headed back to New Jersey for more voice therapy.

I preached a little over the next two years, but for the most part I decided to stay in therapy as long as was necessary. Week after week turned into month after month, but now I could ask for the toll receipt on my own. As a matter of fact, I could do a lot of things that, two years earlier were out of the question. I could now sing hymns

Good Vibrations

at church, I could talk on the phone, and I did not fear a crowd anymore. My voice was getting better.

After three years of lessons, in August 2008, I headed back out to preach and my voice did very well. In my teacher's words, "It held!" Even though I was inconsistent on working it faithfully, it did very well. Often, people commented that they could not believe how well my voice sounded. This was always a great encouragement.

In March of 2009, I returned for additional work and strengthening. For six weeks I did more therapy and she again greatly helped me. The lower end of my voice had begun to strengthen. It had frustrated me that the part of my voice that I use and need most is the last part to "come in". Be that as it was, it is a joy to have a voice now. I know there is more work to be done as it is not 100% yet, but it is very useable now.

When I began voice rehab I was told that my voice was 80% collapsed. Today my voice is well over 80% whole. The best part of it all is that the problem has actually been reversed or healed. This is not a "Band-Aid" that has been applied, but a reversal of the problem, and a correcting of what was wrong.

No, it is not a quick fix, and in this "instant" society, people will often be impatient with such a "cure" as this. But it does work, and I am living proof of that. When I went to the University of

My Story

Pittsburgh Medical Center, they told me that speech therapy would not work, and that my problem was not due to my preaching. They told me to go ahead and preach for I was not hurting my voice. With all due respect I must say that they were 180 degrees off. I believe it was the preaching that caused my trouble.

With regard to speech therapy, they were correct. Speech therapy would not help me at all, for I could not speak. I had no voice. I did not need therapy for my speech. What I needed was physical therapy for the physical instrument in my throat that creates sound. That instrument was not working.

I am not saying, "Don't go to doctors," but the Smolover method of Vocal Behavior Training has corrected my voice problem. If I continue to practice the exercises, my voice will likely become stronger and better than it ever has been in my life. This is very exciting!

I thank my Lord and Saviour Jesus Christ for guiding me to the correct help in restoring my voice.

You can make a story your own, of how you had your voice restored! Yes, if you do the work (and it is going to be work), you will have your own story. It is going to take determination, and more so since you do not have a personal coach like I did. But I am guessing your desire to get your voice back will motivate you to keep at it.

Good Vibrations

    The Smolover method works. This book is about what I did. The one qualifier that I was asked and had to determine was if my vocal ligament had any damage. Damage can be from laser surgery, physical trauma, or a birth defect. If thre is no damage to the ligament then it was likely that I could get my voice back by doing these exercises.

2

Some Things You Should Know

The best way for me to apply the Smolover method was to have a personal instructor guide me through the workouts. I abandoned my preaching schedule and moved where I could visit my teacher's studio twice a week for three years (excluding my brief attempt to get out too soon). Your circumstances may not allow for that; hence, one of the purposes for this book. I will attempt to explain the exercises, as well as the "why" behind them, what I went through as I proceeded, and how I worked my voice toward full rehabilitation.

Through experience I can say that the Smolover method works, but it is work to perform, especially the first year. The only qualification

Good Vibrations

told to me was that if there was something physically wrong with my vocal ligament. If it had been cut, for example, or some other physical impairment was the cause. But I had already gone to a doctor and had a thorough diagnosis performed.

As I mentioned earlier, one of the things that amazed me is when I first talked to my teacher on the phone, in two minutes she told me I had Spasmodic Dysphonia. I replied, *"Yes, that is what they have told me."* I then asked her if she could help me. Without any hesitation whatsoever she replied, *"I know I can. I have helped men get their voice back who have worked on the floor of the New York Stock Exchange."* Her confidence was a great comfort to me.

Let me stress right here that these exercises are work. Like working out at a gym, these exercises are going to be physically working the voice. It is also like learning to walk again. There will be much effort exerted to take what may seem like a little baby step. But as I added step by step I began to walk . . . I began to talk again.

Another thing I would like to stress is that this is not a quick fix. I was told it was going to take time and effort. If I wanted a quick "fix" I could try Botox, though it actually fixes nothing. If I wanted to correct my voice and rehabilitate it, then it was going to take time and steady work. Some people respond quicker than others, but I just had to accept my voice where it was and faithfully do the exercises until it got better.

When I first came to the studio the teacher listened to my voice and told me that my ligament was 80% collapsed. I could make sound on about seven notes in the middle of the piano keyboard. Of those seven notes, only two or three were clear sound. At that time she told me that it would take five years to get my voice back to normal.

This did not deter me. I was just glad to hear that I would get my voice back. Of course "normal" is the goal, but "functional" came much sooner. In fact, I have not been doing my exercises for about a year and a half now because I can function fine the way I am, but at times you can tell my voice is not all the way normal. I really need to do my exercises.

Trying to prepare me, it was also stressed to me what is normal when you do these exercises, but can cause a great deal of fear in you if you are not aware of it. My voice was going to go through changes as it healed. A healing change will start and your voice will actually sound worse. I was told to not be alarmed. It is all part of the process. As I continued to work through the change, my voice would come in stronger and clearer than it was before the change began. I will explain what is happening when I get to the explanation of extrinsic and intrinsic tension.

Consequently, about two months into my

Good Vibrations

therapy my voice began to get worse. (I did not think it possible!) In my mind I began to panic. I thought to myself, *"This lady is ruining what little voice I have left. What am I going to do when I don't have a voice at all?"* And so this fear gripped me, but I had nowhere else to go and nothing else I could do. I just had to keep going.

Then my voice would come in and it would be better than before the change. Oh, what excitement! My voice was getting better and stronger. Instead of seven notes on the piano keyboard, I now had twelve notes that I could make sound on. I was moving in the right direction, but keep in mind, this was after four months of twice-a-week lessons and four additional days of the week spent doing the exercises on my own.

Along with the therapy I would try the Atkins Diet, or stop eating chocolate and any other perceptions of what I could do to help my voice get

---

Voice therapy is useless if the patient refuses to implement the new skills outside the clinic.

In fact, a study led by Verdolini comparing LMRVT (Lessac Madsen Resonant Voice Therapy) to "confidential voice therapy" strongly indicated that patient compliance was a better indicator of therapy effectiveness than the type of therapy administered.[2]

Some Things You Should Know

better. I would come in and tell my teacher the things I was trying, and she would look at me and say, *"The problem is your ligament. A strong ligament will correct all of that. Let's go!"* She would hit the first note and the work would begin.

I also remember, that as I started the work, it would feel as if my voice was all messed up with mucous. I would constantly be clearing my throat, and some of it was mucous. My teacher explained that, when your ligament gets strong it will move the mucous out of the way. This astonished me, but now that my voice is stronger the mucous is not much of a problem at all. The ligament has the strength to work in spite of it, and the sensation was not really mucous at all but the weakness of my ligament.

Something else she told me that I did not believe at the time (but have since found it to be true) was that, as your ligament gets strong, you won't become hoarse when you get sick. I did not believe her, for whenever I got sick the first thing to go (and the last thing to return) was my voice. Now that my ligament is much stronger I do not get hoarse when I am sick like I did before.

Your ligament does not get blood, so it does not get inflamed. It is unaffected by a sore throat.

WHAT I NEEDED:

I was instructed that I needed a quiet room where I could work my voice by myself. I had to

Good Vibrations

be able to concentrate on what I was doing without distraction.

I would also need a piano or a piano keyboard. I could use a half or less keyboard with a computer, but at the start a full-sized keyboard was best.

One more thing; I needed to have a box of tissues handy.

I hope the following story does not cause any fear in you, but I remember coming into the voice studio. It was an average-sized room with a couple of nice chairs at the front window. Then in the middle of the room was about a six-foot grand piano with a couch behind it. Two chairs were by the front of the piano; one for the student and one at the keyboard where the teacher sat in order to play the notes for the student to hum.

I sat down at the student's chair, and my teacher came over with a box of tissues and set them on the edge of the piano in front of me. My teacher was not tall, being about 5' 2". She was in her eighties and wore glasses. Looking at me, she set the tissues on the piano. Then this lady (who I did not really know) smiled and said in a gentle voice, *"I will make you cry."* I was puzzled at this statement, and it must have shown on my face, for she repeated herself, saying again, *"I will make you cry."*

She then proceeded to "work my voice." The first few notes were not bad, but as she went higher and higher up the keyboard, I began to choke as I tried to hum the notes. After a few notes higher, I was straining, grimmacing and do all I could to make sound when tears began to come out of my eyes and she said, *"I told you, I will make you cry."*

Week after week I would go in for therapy and she would work my voice, first with extones and then intones. I would choke, and as I choked and coughed she would say gently, *"I know it's hard, but we have to wake up your ligament. We have to wake it up."* And so the workout would proceed.

As I worked my voice, I was assured that I was not going to hurt it. Then I was reminded that, it may sound a little worse before it gets better. As the change "comes in" my voice would be a little better.

Good Vibrations

3

The Three Modalities

    The exercises that I am writing about in this book are based upon the Smolover method of voice development. They were originally used for singers, but have been found to work in restoring voices to a healthy condition.
    I am going to assume that your voice is not in a healthy condition. Maybe you have Spasmodic Dysphonia Abductor or Adductor. Maybe you have other problems. I am not a doctor, and you should go to a proper voice doctor to find out just exactly what is wrong with your voice. I am only writing about what worked for me. If you have cancer of the vocal cords, or if you have nodules, polyps or other problems, you need to get to a medical doctor.
    On the next couple of pages are some illustrations to hopefully give you an idea of what I am trying to describe.

Good Vibrations

Vocal Fold Lesions

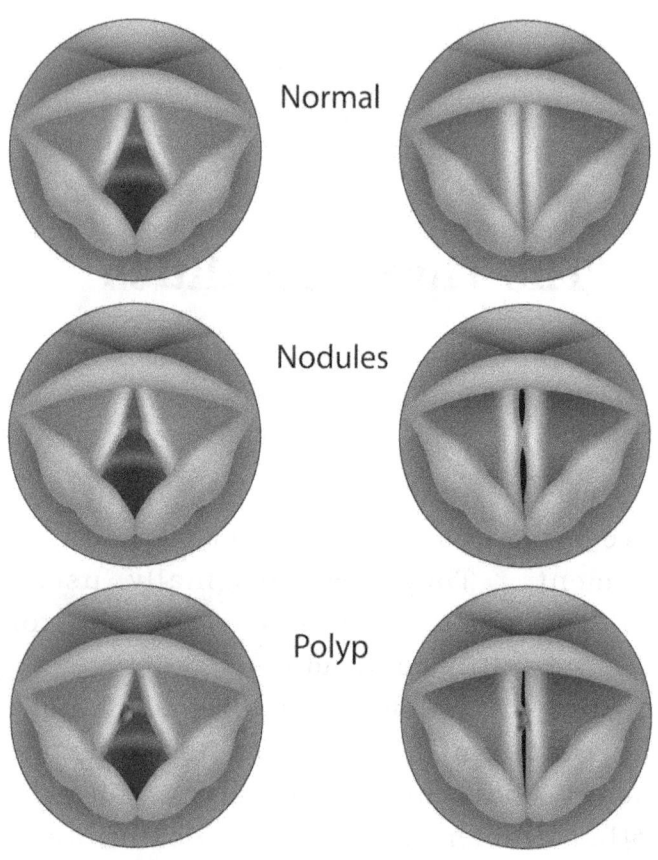

Normal

Nodules

Polyp

Covering each vocal cord is a mucous membrane lining (a moist layer of tissue). Maintaining the health of this lining is essential to your vocal well being. This membrane is called the Vocal Fold. Smoking is very hard on it.[3]

The Three Modalities

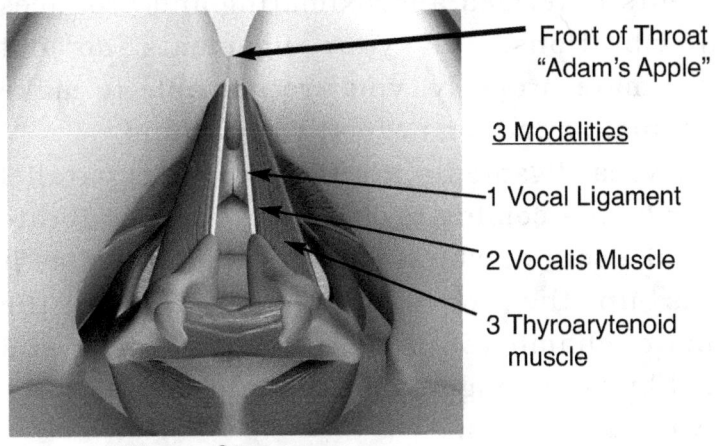

View of Larynx

IMPORTANT - MODALITY ONE - LIGAMENT:

Number one is your ligament. That is the only part of your voice that makes sound by vibrating. Let me write that again, your ligament is the only part of your larynx that makes vibrational sound, and to be more specific, the very edge of your ligaments are the very place where your sound is born.

Modality One is actually two ligaments side by side, with each one being about an eighth of an inch wide. You can see them in the illustration. They separate when you breath, and when you speak they are pushed together as the air travels up between them, being pushed out from your lungs causing them to vibrate, thus making sound. The coming together of the vocal

Good Vibrations

ligaments is termed approximating and produces good vibrations. If your ligaments do not approximate properly, you are not able to make vibrational sound, or normal vocal sound.

Your vocal ligaments are like two taut, parallel rubber bands coming together in order to vibrate and make sound, which is then transformed as it travels up the vocal tract and through the resonate chambers. It is further formed and guided by your tongue and lips into words, notes and various sounds.

Here is Dr. Smolover's description:

> "Each vocal cord is composed of three parallel lengthwise segments. On the inner edge of each cord is the vocal ligament. Next to the vocal ligament is the vocalis muscle, and next to the vocalis is the thyroarytenoid muscle."[3]

These three segments are used in order for you to make vibrational sound. The term for these three segments is modalities. There are three modalities of your voice that we will be dealing with. Each one has a distinct sound, but mainly we will deal with Modality One, the ligament. Modality Two is the vocalis muscle, and Modality Three is the thyroarytenoid muscle.

When your voice functions correctly (and you don't need extra volume), the ligaments come together, or approximate, and make sound. If you

The Three Modalities

need a little more volume, then you call upon the muscle right next to the ligament, which is the vocalis muscle. If you need a lot of volume, you add to the efforts of the ligament and the vocalis muscle, the thyroarytenoid muscle thus creating a very loud sound, or voice. But the whole foundation of your voice rests upon your ligament. If your ligament is not approximating correctly you can call on the vocalis and the thyroarytenoid muscles all you want, but there will be no sound. Why is that?

Because muscle cannot make sound; only your ligament can make sound. That is why much of the Smolover method is comprised of exercises designed to influence your vocal ligament. Get that right, and you have a voice. If it is not right, you will not have a voice.

You will notice that your larynx consists of muscles and ligaments. That is where your voice is created. Well, when your body gets out of shape, don't you have problems? For example, if you pull a muscle or pull a ligament, don't you have trouble? Sometimes it takes merely rest for it to heal, and other times it takes therapy. If you are dealing with the same tissues in your voice, why would it be any different? This is at the heart of the Smolover method.

As I read Connie Pike's latest book, *Free to Speak II: Successful Long Term Management of Spasmodic Dysphonia*, she mentioned that most

Good Vibrations

Spasmodics are people who use their voice a lot, or people who like to talk. I know that is true with me, for I am a preacher. Many people who use their bodies in repetitive ways will often times end up with physical problems resulting from overuse.

I know a man who worked as a train conductor and was always leaning out the window of the locomotive. His back is all messed up from years of doing that. No, his back was not superior in strength because of repetitive use. He has trouble with it.

How many athletes intensively use their bodies for a while and then are unable to continue due to the problems arising from the amount of use or the repetitive motions of the activities in which they perform? Their problems are not due to faulty nerves, or faulty brain signals. Their problems are due to overuse.

Having said that, though, there are other people with physical problems just because of the body they have. They also need physical therapy to heal, or to restore as much as possible the function of their body. If you are out of shape physically, then it takes time, effort, and the proper exercises to get the muscles and ligaments back to the strength they need to be.

One man said to his wife, after she was harping on him about his weight, *"I am in shape; round is a shape!"* That wasn't quite what she had in mind.

The Three Modalities

So too is the theory behind the Smolover method, also known as Vocal Behavior Training or VBT. If your voice is not working correctly, here are some exercises to get it back in shape so it will work correctly and you will be able to talk, speak, sing, yell, or whatever you want to do with your voice. It has taken fifty years for these exercises to be developed.

At the root of the problem is your ligament because it is your ligament that makes sound. Ligaments take longer to heal. A ligament takes

---

Physical Therapy For The Voice

Once "warmed," the singer may proceed to daily exercises. The work of Sabol, Lee, & Stemple (1995) explains that many of the exercises prescribed for vocal flexibility are actually calisthenic exercises.

Vocal Function Exercises, first described by Barnes and modified by Dr. Joseph Stemple, are "a series of direct, systematic voice manipulations (exercises), similar in theory to physical therapy for the vocal folds, designed to strengthen and balance the laryngeal musculature, and to improve the efficiency of the relationship among airflow, vocal fold vibration, and supraglottic treatment of phonation."[4]

time to heal because a ligament does not get blood directly. A muscle will heal faster due to the blood flow through it, but a ligament is not that way; it takes longer. Therefore the Smolover method is not a quick fix. It takes time and work, but it corrects what is wrong. The Smolover method is not a bandage. It is vocal rehabilitation of your ligament and the surrounding muscles to get them back into the shape they need to be for proper operation.

When I read about the treatments at various spasmodic clinics I understand what they are doing, and why it is so quick, but they are not fixing anything. Let me explain.

The two ligaments vibrating together make vocal sound. As your voice rises higher in pitch your ligaments come together and vibrate at a different position than they do when you make sound at a lower pitch. Not only that, but the ligament narrows for higher pitch and becomes thicker for lower pitch. Think of the strings of a piano and you will kind of get the idea of what I am talking about: thinner strings for higher sounds, and thicker strings make the lower sounds.

When you talk, you talk at a certain pitch. If you get excited then the pitch may raise a little, or if you are tired or relaxed it may lower a little. But for the most part, when you talk, you always talk at about the same pitch. So that spot on your ligament is used the most. And if you talk a

The Three Modalities

lot, that particular spot on your ligament is used a lot. Now, let's say that spot, or position, of your ligament gets weak, tired, or stretched for whatever reason. Overuse? Possibly, but that is not always the case. Nevertheless, it is not working as it should, but there are other positions on your ligament that have not been used so much and are in good shape.

If you can raise the pitch of sound and move to a new location on your ligament (one which is not worn out and is working properly) then your problem seems to go away. You are at a new spot on your ligament, so it works to make sound. If the new spot is above your worn out spot then you will have to raise the pitch of your voice so as to use a new place on your vocal ligament. If the spot you want to use is lower, then you will have to lower the pitch of your voice so as to use that spot on your vocal ligament.

These other SD rehab clinics are merely directing people to raise or lower their voice pitch so as to use a different part of their vocal ligament. They are not curing, or rehabilitating, the worn out spot. They are merely finding a new spot on the ligament to use, or as Connie Pike says, "Your new groove."

She mentions, though, that sometimes you can slip back into your old groove, which means your voice does not work right. You have gone back down to that old part of the ligament that didn't work before. Your ligament, or your Spasmodic Dysphonia has not been corrected at all. You have just gone to a different spot on your ligament. If that spot becomes weak, then you will have to find another and learn to talk there. But in all of this hunting and searching for your new voice nothing has been corrected or repaired.

The Smolover method is not that way. The Smolover method is a set of exercises designed to work and rehabilitate your vocal ligament and the surrounding muscles so that they work as a team like they are designed to do in order to make sound. This method corrects what is wrong with your voice, but it takes work, time and effort.

I want also to say, that if you have been helped by Connie Pike, Dr. Cooper, or anyone else, I am happy for you. If you have been helped and your voice is restored, I am glad for you. I am not trying to say one way is right or wrong. The goal is to help people get their voices restored.

I was reading testimonies in Connie Pike's second book and came across the testimony of a man who is a pastor. He also came to the teacher I used. I remember him. He had SD and went to a couple of spasmodic clinics for help. He then came to my teacher while I was in my second year of therapy. For the sake of space I will not quote the whole testimony, but after many different treatments and therapies to restore his voice, this is what is recorded in her book:

The Three Modalities

"In March 2006, he began working with a singing teacher, _____, who had recovered from SD herself. She used the Smolover method with him for four months. **His voice returned**, (emphasis added) but he continued to feel effort in voicing and breathing."[5]

He responded excellently to the therapy and, in only four months, his voice was extremely improved. It was my teacher and the Smolover method that worked for him.

If one part, or position, of your ligament is not working properly, and you then move up above or down below that position on the ligament, you can find a place that may still function. Your voice will operate at a different pitch, but you have cured nothing. It may seem like a quick fix, and for many they are content with the results they get. There is nothing wrong with that. Just understand that nothing has been corrected or fixed; the weakness is still there.

The design of the Smolover method is to rehabilitate the ligament as well as the muscles. It is a correction of the problem.

Good Vibrations

I found the following quote encrouraging:

However, a study using Lindquest's technique and exercises produced **positive therapeutic results** for singers with pathology such as hyperfunction, nodules, **paralyzed vocal fold**, and iatrogenic complications. Evidently, the exercises did not put undue strain on the already hyperfunctional and/or physiologically abnormal voice, but **the benefits of exercise for a healthy larynx held true for the pathological voice.** Therapy using the Lindquest exercise routine has continued for over fifteen years, producing similar results. Thus, appropriately designed and executed exercises have the potential to train and develop the voice and to help maintain and *restore vocal health.*[6]

4

Practical Tips For Voice

Chances are if you have SD you have already tried these tips, but there may be some who are reading this book whose voice is normal and they are just wanting to strengthen it, or help it get even better. This method of vocal working and strengthening is not just for those who suffer from SD. These exercises are for anyone who wants to improve their voice.

Dr. Smolover originally designed these exercises for singers and performers on stage. The benefit for those of us with SD is that these exercises will also work for voice restoration.

A strong ligament will do much to eliminate voice problems for it is the ligament that actually makes the sound. Your ligament is surrounded by muscle, but muscle cannot make sound. Here are

Good Vibrations

some practical recommendations for your voice that can help, and when ignored, can greatly hinder you from having a voice.

The first tip is rest. If you have a weak voice, the weakest link will break when you are tired, and that will be your voice. Make sure that you are rested. When my voice started getting rough, I would come home for a few weeks and within a week it was like new. As my voice got worse then it would take two weeks and then a month, but eventually it would never recover, even after four months of Doctor-prescribed rest with no talking. If you are not that bad, then rest may greatly help you.

The second tip is to make sure that your body is hydrated. By that I mean that you are not dehydrated. In terms of performers, I believe the admonition is that you are to have "pale pee". This is very important. Water is your voice's best friend. Make sure you are well hydrated when you are getting ready to use your voice, and make sure you are well hydrated when you are getting ready to work your voice. It will greatly help.

Caffeine, salt, and other foods that dehydrate you should be avoided prior to a workout, or you should compensate by drinking an extra amount of water.

The third tip is if you are speaking in public get a Public Address system that works! One of my biggest complaints about the churches that I go

Practical Tips For Voice

to for meetings is that it is common for them to not have an adequate sound system. Then those that do have an adequate sound system, often times don't properly use it. This frustrates me to no end.

If people have left their busy schedules to come out to a meeting, they ought to be able to hear you. That is the whole purpose of the meeting. I remember speaking in a church that was modern and had a very good sound system. They actually had the sound system turned off. A man who was visiting that evening mentioned to me that he could not hear the pastor at the beginning of the service. He could hear me for I had brought my own sound system. I was incredulous at the obvious lack of cognizance of the need for his voice to be amplified. If someone comes to a meeting and can't hear, they certainly are not coming back. People appreciate the ability to hear for that is why they left their home. Get a sound system and use it!

I have my own portable sound system. It is a Bose L1 compact with a Sennheiser EW 122 G3 series cordless microphone. This is an amazing system and will easily reach a crowd of 300, and possibly 500 depending on the room.

Maybe you are not a public speaker. You are just someone who wants to get his voice back. Your voice will return if you do the work. But if necessary, there are such things as personal PA

Good Vibrations

systems that are small and suitable for amplifying your voice. It may seem strange but they do work well. Until your voice gets strong you may need to check into this. BHphotovideo.com has some of these if you are interested in a starting reference of where to look.

Spasmodic clinics often stress breathing and calmness because when you're tense, your voice will have a tendency to disappear. The breathing trains you to stay calm. A PA system has a way of doing that same thing even better.

Of course the other reason they teach breathing and staying calm is because they are not strengthening your voice, but merely finding another place on your vocal ligament that will vibrate. This may help temporarily, but your ligament is still weak.

> **Water**
>
> **Specifically, adequate hydration can help to minimize the effects of phonotrauma.**
>
> **Hydration also reduces the lung pressure required for vocal fold oscillation, which the patient recognizes as decreased effort.[2]**

5

What Are You Doing?

Your vocal sound is made by the ligament, Modality One, coming together, also known as approximating. In order for sound to be made the ligament, Modality One, must be aligned, strong, and flexible. In the next chapter are exercises to get your ligament into shape so as to be aligned, flexible, strong, and operating freely without having to use extrinsic tension.

EXTRINSIC AND INTRINSIC TENSION:

Extrinsic tension is the enemy of your voice. A cripple may have one weak leg, but in order to walk he uses his other leg more and relies on it more. The healthy leg becomes very strong so as

Good Vibrations

to make up for the weakness of the other leg. This is a simple explanation of what happens when your voice becomes weak. For a man or woman to strengthen the good leg is a good thing, but for you to build up strength from other parts of your body to make up for your vocal weakness is not a good thing. It actually becomes a hindrance.

As your voice became weak you attempted to compensate for the weakness by propping it up with crutches, so to speak. Maybe you had to push just a bit harder, or you called on muscles in your neck, jaw, shoulders, or perhaps your whole body in order to hit a certain pitch, or to simply make sound. As your vocal ligament continued to weaken, you called upon muscles outside of your larynx to help you make the sound, and these muscles, though needed at the time, have come to hinder your voice. They may be overriding your larynx. Now what is needed is for your larynx to strengthen, especially your vocal ligament. Your ligament needs to have the strength to stand on its own, without any help, and for those extrinsic helpers to back down.

You may wonder, if I used "helpers" in order to compensate for my weakness, and now my voice is very weak, how will I ever be able to back off from these outside muscles, or what we refer to as extrinsic tension, i.e. muscles outside of the larynx?

What Are You Doing?

You will do it inch by inch. Tiny by tiny, little baby steps at first. This is one of the reasons you must relax and be in a quiet, distraction-free room.

When I first started working my voice I would pull my head to my right side. Why? I don't know. It just seemed to help me make sound. I would grimace, tighten my neck, clench my fists, close my eyes, lean over, twist, and so on, all for the purpose of trying to make sound. I am not exaggerating. My voice was gone! These were all forms of extrinsic tension.

When your ligament is working freely, in conjunction with the muscles along side it, then your voice is just there. Pavarotti, Sinatra, Streisand and others make it look easy when they sing. Their voices are just there. Sound seems to flow out effortlessly. Such performers have a very well developed and healthy ligament, thus eliminating extrinsic tension. Their voices are "free".

Intrinsic tension is the tension formed from within the larynx. When your voice is operating properly, that is all the muscle and help your ligament will call upon, and it is all that you will need in order to make sound. Modalities One, Two and Three will be all you need and will bear up for whatever you call upon them to do, within reason.

Good Vibrations

VOCAL CHANGES OR TRANSITIONS:

At the end of Chapter 2, I mentioned that your voice might sound worse before it gets better. Let me explain.

I just mentioned the need for your extrinsic tension to back off and let your ligament stand on its own. As you do these exercises, that is exactly what is going to happen, but if you are not aware of it you may get a bit concerned or fearful that your voice is getting worse. Here is what happens:

These exercises are designed to work the intrinsic muscles and ligaments of your larynx, with the great majority of the work focused on your ligament, Modality One. As you work your ligament it starts to grow and become stronger, but the work you are doing bypasses the extrinsic "helpers" that you have been using to prop up your voice in order to make sound.

As your ligament grows stronger the extrinsic helpers begin to die out, little by little. You could say that the various crutches you have been using to prop up your voice are going to be kicked out one by one.

As each little crutch gets kicked out, your voice kind of stands there and wobbles for a little while. You could say it is a bit shaky on its feet. Then, after a week or so, it increases its strength to bear up a little more on its own. As it does, your voice comes back in a little bit stronger than it was before the change.

This process of the extrinsic helpers dying out and the intrinsic strength coming in and growing takes place over and over as your voice returns to its full strength, and even better than ever.

THE EXERCISES:

This is what I was instructed to do.

These exercises preferably should be done by sitting at a piano or full-sized keyboard, while softly humming on pitch as best you can, with your mouth closed as you strike each note.

For a voice that is very bad (as mine was) then at the beginning the person is just going to have to make sound any way they can. For Adductor SD relax and try to hum a very soft, clear and what we call "tiny" sound. If you start to tense, then stop, relax and take your time. Later you will keep moving, but this is for the very beginning of your rehab. For Abductor SD relaxing may be difficult, but still try for soft, clear and tiny sound. Some notes will be easier than others.

When I choked sometimes it would be a couple of minutes before I was ready to move to the next note. I had to remember, "This is work! It was not necessarily going to be fun."

Good Vibrations

Tiny and Small Sound

VERY IMPORTANT: I was told that when I worked my voice the sound I was to make was to be tiny and small. I was concentrating work on my ligament and, to be specific, the very edge of my ligament for it is the very edge of the ligament that makes all of the sound. By working the very edge of the ligament I was rehabilitating my voice from the inside out. Starting at the very edge a person will begin to restore the function of the ligament, then strengthen it and in so doing cause the extrinsic "helpers" to cease because they are no longer needed.

Doctors claim that because of the involuntary spams of the nerves you cannot control what the very edge of your ligament does, and to some extent that may be true. That is what they told me. But what I needed to do was to find the part

> LMRVT is unique in that it corrects both hypo- and hyperadducted vocal fold posturing by guiding vocal behavior toward **barely-abducted** or **barely-adducted** laryngeal posturing.[2]
>
> Exercise #1: Thin Edge Function
> Perform the following exercise using the image that you are going to **barely touch the finest edge of the vocal folds**.[7]

What Are You Doing?

of my ligament that still worked and little by little, AS MY LIGAMENT STRENGTHENED I would gain control. My voice was out of control because of a weak, misaligned, or stiff ligament.

I know I am repeating myself but, I was to work the very edge of my ligament; therefore, the sound is to be tiny. I was to slowly bring the vocal chords together and just as they began to make sound stay right there.

It is similar to the Vocal Function exercises recommended by Stemple or Lessac. The difference with Smolover is that the exercises are performed with your mouth closed. They are done as a hum. This is to direct the effort to the ligament and removes extrinsic tension from the jaw.

My instructor, was an opera singer in New Jersey, just across the Hudson River from Broadway. After years of telling her to push the voice and to push harder (thinking it would strengthen), she eventually lost her voice. Dr. Smolover called her one day and asked her how she was doing, and she hoarsely told him that she could no longer sing. She had worked with him already on a study of voice at the University of New York City, and they were acquainted through music chorales as well.

So, he asked her if she would be willing to work with him to find out how to get her voice back, and she agreed. She told me that for the first ten

Good Vibrations

years they had no idea of what to do. They experimented with various ways of placing the tongue, or mouth position and other things. Then one day, after more than ten years of probing and searching, she said Dr. Smolover, an Orthodox Jew, came into his New York City office where she was waiting to start a new voice lesson and said to her, "I have been so stupid."

Astonished, she looked at him and asked, "Why?"

He replied, "Because it is not in the push that you are going to get strength. It is in the still small voice." So they began a new method of working the human voice, which was to work it with a tiny, small sound. Year after year they worked and worked. When I came to my teacher for voice lessons she had been working with Dr. Smolover for over forty years.

I was instructed to attempt to make a clear small sound at each note. At first this may be impossible. As I started out, I had to make sound any way I could, and it was hard. Little by little (after six months or so), I was able to back off, and the sound would become clear and small.

For Adductor SD, (when the vocal chords are tightly closed) this may not be the case, and the only way to make sound is to relax and start very, very small and get it to grow. Either way, the goal is a tiny voice that works the edge of your ligament.

What Are You Doing?

STRETCH:

Have you ever done stretching exercises? Some people are limber. But others, like me, are not. I hate stretching exercises, but I need to do them. So too it is with your voice. When you are young, it is much easier to stretch because you are more limber. As you get older, if you have been stretching all your life, it is no problem to stretch. If you have not been stretching all your life, to begin stretching at 40, 50, or 60 years old is a challenge, but it needs to be done. This is true with your voice, as well. I was told to stretch my ligament in order to get it limber, and to help align it. I'll write about alignment next.

I was to hum notes in ascending order, going up the piano keyboard, obviously the pitch becomes higher and higher. As I made the sounds higher and higher, my ligament has stretching in order to make the approximation and thus create sound. The ligament becomes smaller and thinner as the notes get higher and higher. This became stretching work out.

ALIGNMENT:

To make sound two ligaments must approximate, or come together equally, as the air

Good Vibrations

passes between them causing them to vibrate. In order to do this not only do the ligaments need to be flexible and strong, but they must also be aligned side-by-side or there will be no vibration. As a person vocally ascends higher and higher on the scale, the ligament (Modality One) is fine-tuned, you might say, and aligned. Then, from the top a person begins to bring it down so the alignment meets all the way down the edge of your ligament. To bring the alignment down takes months of daily work, but is essential for sound to be made.

FLEX:

Your ligament must also be flexible. Vibration is a fast flexing of the very edge of your ligament. In order to get my ligament flexible I would not only be doing extones, which is humming outward, but I would also learn to do intones, which is humming inward. Intones are not easy to do!

As you exhale, air is pushed up and out between the ligament, making an extone. The vocal ligament flexes up due to the movement of air coming from your lungs as you exhale. This occurs with normal speaking.

Intone is much more difficult, but is very good for Spasmodic Dysphonia. Intones are very

What Are You Doing?

important, especially if you are Spasmodic.

> "Intoning is a feature of some spoken languages and has been used effectively in voice therapy for conditions such as spasmodic dysphonia, a vocal disorder in which laryngeal spasm prevents normal speech."[8]

Dr. Gartner-Schmidt at UPMC told me that intoning was a great exercise and very helpful for Spasmodic Dysphonia.

When a person intones they are drawing air down thier throat and through their larynx, thus causing the ligament to flex in the opposite direction. Sounds simple, doesn't it? Wait until you try it! Chances are your ligament is not used to doing this. With practice it will get better, but there will likely be a certain amount of ...choking and coughing!

WHY DO I CHOKE?

Muscle does not (cannot) make or create sound. Only your ligament makes sound, but your ligament does not need muscle to make sound. The ligament can make sound all by itself, which is one of the characteristics of a healthy ligament. If you need more volume you can call on the

Good Vibrations

vocalis muscle (Modality Two), which is positioned right next to your ligament. If you need even more volume, you can call on the thyroarytenoid muscle (Modality Three).

    A familiar explanation of when sound is created from ligament only is what is termed the falsetto. The Bee Gees sang in this manner and some of the harmonics of the Beach Boys used this as well. Often it is attributed to male singers, but it actually applies to both male and female voices. Modality One (ligament only) is a high sounding function. When the vocalis muscle beside your ligament (Modality Two) is used it sounds basically normal, like regular speaking or singing, and is lower in pitch. When the thyroarytenoid muscle (Modality Three) is called upon for help, you may think of it as a man singing opera with a big, deep, loud voice.

    When your ligament is weak, you bring it together in order to make sound as usual. But if the ligament cannot bear up under the pressure of being pushed together, it will begin to collapse or roll over. Remember, your ligament has no feeling, for there are no nerves going to it, but the muscle does contain nerves and has feeling. As your ligament collapses or rolls over, the muscles from each side of your voice box begin to touch. When they touch, there is stimulation to those nerves in those muscles because they are now rubbing together. This sensation is felt and

What Are You Doing?

causes you to choke, cough, and even get close to passing out. I write from experience for this has happened to me many times, and still does, when I work my voice vigorously.

As a ligament becomes strong it is able to bear up under the pressure that it is being called upon to handle in order to make the sound. Thus, the choking stops and sound is born.

I was diagnosed with Abductor SD, which meant that my ligament was not coming together in order to make sound. I would try to talk but the air would pass right through with little or no vibration of the ligament. I think my ligament was just blowing apart like two worn out rubber bands! It had no strength to hold together and, therefore, could not vibrate. They would blow apart or, in medical terminology, they would "abduct."

The medical theory was that the nerves going to Modalities Two and Three were overactive. They were giving too strong of a signal so the muscles were contracting and thus pulling the ligament apart. Whether that was so or not, I don't know. I do know that my voice is working now.

Maybe the exercises have restored enough strength to my ligament that the nerves, while still giving the same amount of pull, are not causing the ligament to abduct. I am not a doctor, so this is only a theory, but I do know that my voice is now working so that I can talk, speak

Good Vibrations

and sing.

I also know that "Ad-" ductor SD is the opposite of "Ab-" ductor SD. With Adductor SD, the vocal ligament becomes closed off so that no air can pass between the ligaments. Again, I'm only theorizing, but this sounds to me as if the ligament is not aligned and may be overlapping. If that is the case, then when the air comes up, the pressure of the breath closes the overlapping ligaments, thus restricting the movement of air. This would create a sensation of choking. To me it seems like the ligament is mis-aligned. Perhaps the ligament is slammed together so tight air does not pass through.

If the ligament can be strengthened so that it does not collapse when it is approximated, then this condition will be alleviated. With a strong and aligned ligament the very edge of the ligament will be able to vibrate, allowing the air to pass through under control. My teacher had tremendous success with Adductor Spasmodics.

NODULES, POLYPS, AND OTHER PROBLEMS:

In my last months with my teacher she had a professional female singer come to her with the diagnosis of nodes on her vocal cords. Nodes, simply put, are calluses on the vocal cord that make the very edge of the ligament uneven,

What Are You Doing?

partially abducted and hard to vibrate. They happen due to uneven pressure being placed on the cord when sound is made, thus rubbing and causing a callus to form. The standard prescription is to cease talking for a few months, but that does not fix the problem of unequal pressure being exerted on different parts of the ligament.

While it may be true that if you have calluses on your hands and you quit doing rough work, the calluses will go away, such is not the case with nodes on the vocal cords.

My teacher worked with this singer who had been told she needed to have the nodes surgically removed. The surgery is very dangerous to the voice and can ruin it if not properly done. One mistake by the surgeon, and your voice may be permanently damaged, or even lost. That is what happened to Julie Andrews.[9]

By working with the lady and doing the exercises, in less than a year the nodes were gone. The voice doctor she was going to was exceedingly astonished.

Here is another testimony of someone being helped or healed through voice exercises:

> This soprano was referred to my (David Jones) studio by her voice therapist. Frustrated from her past performances at the Metropolotan

Opera, she was suffering from imbalance in registration, which had led to pushing a large amount of breath pressure through the larynx. She also suffered from edema (swelling) on the right vocal fold.

Her doctor had told her she might be a candidate for surgery. Within the first 10 seconds it was easy to diagnose what was wrong with her voice. Her jaw had developed the habit of thrusting forward.

We adjusted the jaw position back, which was a challenge since the right side of the jaw had come forward out of its socket. Just three months later, she met me in Europe for two sessions. Her first good news was that the edema had disappeared and she no longer needed vocal fold surgery.

The realignment of the vocal folds was due to the realignment of the jaw, which we had accomplished in the New York lessons. This singer has continued her career without vocal problems.[10]

It has been amusing to me to read of the various theories as to how to treat Spasmodic Dysphonia.

What Are You Doing?

Now, I am writing as one who has been diagnosed with Abductor SD, and the Smolover method has worked for me. During my three intensive years with my teacher, unless the ligament was actually broken, every student that came in got their voice back. She even had one lady come to her with asthma. The lady was not trying to be cured of asthma. She was coming to try to learn sing. But after years of voice lessons and work her asthma was gone! The humming and holding your breath is a great work out for your lungs, as well.

What has also been amusing is how some think it is the nerves, or the brain signals, or the breath, etc. But if the instrument is broken, then the instrument needs to be fixed! Yes, I know, I am not a doctor. I am just someone who could not talk and now I can talk and sing.

I am ashamed to admit this, but I have not been doing my exercises regularly now for over five years. Is my voice perfect? Almost, but if I would do my exercises it would get better than it has ever been. The problem is that your voice gets very useable, and then you become so busy you don't take the time to work on it. I say this as one whom, at one time, could not talk. When I say could not talk, that is exactly what I mean. I could not talk on the phone or in public if I had to compete with other noise. It was impossible for me to compete with other noises. I would look to my wife, and, generally, she would know what I was trying to say. I am so thankful to have such a close relationship with my wife.

What I am getting at, though, is that it has been two years since consistently working my voice, and it is holding. This is with semi-forceful public speaking, sometimes from Sunday to Sunday, and it is holding well. What was wrong has been reversed and made right.

JUMP ROPE:

The upper end of my voice came in very well, and then the lower end came in well, but the center of my voice was taking its sweet time. Even now there are a few notes in the middle of my vocal range that are a bit weak. (I just need to be working my voice.)

My voice teacher once suggested that I think of a jump rope, especially when they did doubles, for you have two ligaments. The jump ropes were tightest at the ends, and the middles had the most play. Your voice is like that. The ligament is anchored at the ends, but it will take time for the good behavior to reach all the way to the center. It will eventually, but it just takes time.

Breathy Voicing

In 1969, Fox presented some positive therapy results with a case of spastic dysphonia. Therapy consisted of teaching the patient to speak in a breathy voice **so that the vocal folds would make minimal, if any, contact.** Fox reported that the woman was able to eliminate the tremulous strainded quality 75-80% of the time in daily life. This was the first reported account in the literature of success in reducing spastic symptomatology through therapy. It was ahead of its time in presenting a reduction rather than complete remission of symptoms as successful treatment.[11]

References to the Old Italian School

Technically, Lindquest combined the principles of the Italian school with those gained from the studio of a Swedish throat surgeon, professional singer, and voice teacher...[6]

Proctor also advocates use of exercises similar to those from the Italian school. Examples he gives are an exercise to aid singers in breath control (a prolonged crescendo and diminuendo on a tone sustained as long as possible), a flexibility scale, and scales which work over the "break" or register change in the voice.[6]

6

My First Exercise & Daily Workout

For the first week or maybe two weeks of exercises I only did the extone exercise. It is a simple exercise so it got me used to working my voice.

An extone is performed by taking a deep breath inward, so that you fill your lungs with air, and then with your mouth closed, humming a tiny sound with the air traveling out through your nose.

I was instructed to be in a quiet room by myself with no distractions. My phone was to be turned off and left in another room. I really needed to know that I was not going to be disturbed. I was to be seated in front of a piano or a piano keyboard. I was to be seated upright, not laying back but upright, so that my neck would be straight.

My teacher told me, "As you are seated, stop for a moment, relax and think about how to do your workout. You are going to press the key, and as you hear the sound, you are going to quietly hum the same note. You should hum this note for five counts (or seconds), if possible. Remember to think tiny."

I was told that a tiny voice was one that is made just as you bring the ligaments together. They are to barely touch, and it is better if they don't touch. With as little breath as possible make sound.

This was hard for me because my ligaments were just blowing apart. They had no strength to stay together.

Then she would tell me, "You want to hum and make a tiny, clear sound with your mouth closed, as this will help avoid using any extrinsic tension. As you are making this sound, you are to concentrate on what you are doing. Your tongue should be relaxed and not used to help you make any sound. Don't let your mind wander. At first, that will be easy as it is a new experience. Later, your mind may have a tendency to wander, but try not to let that happen. You need to concentrate on your ligament and the sound that it is making.

I know at first it is all new, but you will come to understand it all by and by.

My First Exercise & Daily Workout

When searching for your "home base," middle C, or C4 is a good place to start. Once you find your range, you should start as low as you are able. Strike the note and hum for five counts. You can tap your toe or foot or something like that for five counts. The length of time does not have to be exact.

As you hum the note, try to relax. Depending upon your condition this will be hard at first. The first weeks, you will make the sound any way you can, and then, in time, as tiny as possible so as to work the edge of your ligament.

And then she would tell me not to try to do these exercises without a keyboard!!! You will not do them correctly."

For example, driving down the road. I was to work my ENTIRE ligament, not just certain sections. I was told that I must use a keyboard, or an instrument that will step by step and note by note ascend and descend the scale. I couldn't have worked my voice anyway while I was driving for I choked so hard I would almost pass out.

Dr. Smolover, in his book, *Sing Your Best*, showed how to use a guitar for the work, but piano is easiest and best.

So, I was now seated at my piano in a quiet, distraction-free room. Relax! I always prayed before I started, for I needed all the help I could get!

She told me, "Hit the first note and determine

Good Vibrations

the lowest note from which you can start. (Don't be afraid. You are not going to make a mistake, but you must start somewhere. This was a comfort to me.) Hum that note for five counts. Remember, tiny and clear, if possible. Do your best. Now strike the next note higher and do the same thing. If you are musical you can do a scale. (I personally ended up just doing all white keys.) Note by note, go as high as you are able. Dr. Smolover used whole steps, but I use scales. It's up to you, she would tell me.

You are stretching your ligament and aligning it, the higher you go.

Once you are as high as you can go, try to go two notes higher. Yes, it is work! S-T-R-E-T-C-H! Rest for a minute and then start again at the highest attempted note and move down the keyboard to as low as you can, sustaining each note for five counts. When you reach your lowest note, try to go two notes lower.

At the bottom of your range, the last two attempts may just be breath with no sound, but try it anyway. In time, it will begin to make sound."

When I started I had no sound below -C2. My breath just fell right through. Now I can sustain a hum for ten counts five notes below -C2, and can make sound at -C3. It took time and effort, Oh boy did it take effort! But my voice did eventually respond.

My First Exercise & Daily Workout

She instructed me, "OK, you just did your first exercise. Rest a bit.

Now do it again. Relax and think tiny; up as high as you can go and then two notes higher. Take a short rest, and then back down to as low as you can go, then two notes lower. Do not hurry! For your first two weeks, your work-out should be extones, five counts up and down the keyboard three times, and that's it."

I was motivated and worked and worked my voice, probably overworking it. The road to recovery was going to take time. I was to be consistent and work my voice for six days and then take one day off.

I was to always end my work-out by descending down the keyboard. This is how I was to bring the ligament down.

SUMMARY OF WORKOUT:

Extone for five counts, up and back down the keyboard, three times. I was to go as high as I could make sound, and then go two notes higher, but tiny. Then I was to always end going down the keyboard to my lowest note, and then go two notes lower.

Good Vibrations

7

2nd Work Out
Third Or Forth Week

My teacher instructed me, "Now you are going to do the same exercise, but you are going to try to sustain the note for twelve counts. You may not be able to at first, but think tiny and clear, and hold for twelve counts, or as long as you are able. Barely bring your ligaments together. Be gentle if you can. Some notes will do better than others. There is nothing you can do about that, it is what it is. Do this three times per workout.

The sustaining of the note builds strength. So now, you are not only stretching your ligament in order to make it limber and able to expand your vocal range, but you are also adding strength. Hum for twelve counts on each note, moving up the keyboard to as high as you can go, and then two notes higher. Take a short rest. Now, back

Good Vibrations

down the keyboard to as low as you can go, and then two notes lower. Yes, it is quite a work-out isn't it? You are just beginning.

ALWAYS END BY GOING DOWN THE KEYBOARD. As you move up, you are using ligament only at the high notes. By coming down the keyboard you are going to be bringing that behavior, which is ligament only, down. Going up high also aligns the ligament at the upper end. By descending the keyboard, you will be bringing this alignment down, thus enabling your ligament to approximate. Little by little, it will come down over time."

I remember her telling me these things over and over.

SUMMARY OF WORKOUT:

I was to extone tiny for twelve counts, or as long as you could, going up the keyboard and then two notes higher. Brief rest, catch my breath, and then from the highest note I was to work down the keyboard, three times. I was to always end going down the keyboard to my lowest note.

8

3rd Workout
Third Month

Each of the first two workouts would serve me well for the first two months. I remember working my voice and some notes I could go twenty counts, and others I could barely go three. My ligament was very unequal in strength, alignment and flexibility. Then she brought in a new exercise. Oh boy, what a time!

This new exercise was added somewhere about the third month and after that, other exercises were to be added much more slowly. Obviously, I did not have immediate access to all of the exercise instructions which are included in this book. I was instructed to move slowly. It may have taken longer than what I am saying here. Each exercise builds on those previous so it took time to move forward.

Good Vibrations

I was intructed to, "Start this work-out by doing the five-count ex-tones as you did in the first weeks. That works your stretch. Next, you are going to work on the flex of your ligament. If you are going to make sound, you have to have a flexible ligament.

Start at your first note and extone for five counts. Now, on the same note, strike the key again, but this time you are going to intone. You are to make sound, tiny if possible, by humming inward with your mouth closed. Hold this note for five counts. At first just make sound any way you can. In time, you will be able to make sound tiny, but at first this may be impossible."

The comfort to me was when she told me that on intones, no matter how you make sound you are not going to hurt your voice. The goal was to just make sound any way you could while breathing inward.

> Intone, counting over 10, ... Intoning is the most fantastic means of releasing the voice into speaking.[12]
>
> "In addition to therapeutic singing, vocal intonation therapy2 can again accomplish the goal of improving voice quality."[13]

Third Workout, Third Month

Intones are performed by emptying your lungs and then, with your mouth closed, humming while drawing air inward into your lungs.

She told me, "There is a possibility that you are going to choke during this exercise. Due to the weakness of the ligament, when it is approximated it may collapse, or roll over, thus allowing the muscles to rub together. The nerves in the muscles respond, causing you to cough and choke. If this happens, just do your best and work through it. (See Chapter 5, What Are You Doing? under, Why Do I Choke? for the complete explanation.)

Little by little, as your ligament strengthens, these so-called "stitches," will become fewer and fewer to non-existent. When the ligament has the strength to stay approximated, it will not roll over. The muscles will not touch anymore, and you will be free from the choking." Oh, how I looked forward to the day I would not choke anymore!

Intoning was very hard for me. I choked and choked on the intoning. I don't wish that on anyone! I remember in the beginning, and for quite a few months, when I would intone upward, there was a point above middle C where it felt to me as if my voice was in one big knot. Obviously, it wasn't, but it felt that way. I would climb the scale intoning with a little difficulty, but not too much. When I approached about +C1, I had a battle on my hands. Well, actually, the battle was

Good Vibrations

in my throat. I just had to work through it; choke, stitch, tears and all. Little by little, after a year or so, it finally broke through and went away, but it was work.

I will try to explain in a way you can understand, but it is very difficult to describe.

When I would make sound in a difficult area of the keyboard, it seemed to be coming from behind this big tangled knot in my vocal chords. The sound seemed to be made behind the knot, and I would have to give it all I had just to get sound to take place. After months of work, there began this tiny little sound in front of that tangled knot. I was told to go for that sound in the front. It was so weak and tiny, delicate, and hard to grab, but one day I was able to make sound in the front of that big tangled knot. The work that I had to do in making sound behind that tangled knot was no longer needed. I could make sound in front of the knot, which was much easier, though not as loud. Little by little, the knot went away.

If I were going to guess, I would say that, for me, right there my ligament was not aligned so as to cause a good amount of interference in the operation of the ligament. My teacher would just say my ligament was weak there.

How often I would analyze my voice, only to have my teacher tell me to just work it, don't analyze it. She would tell me, "You have a weak ligament, and it needs to be worked!

Third Workout, Third Month

Your ligament is not used to flexing in the opposite direction. It may roll over, muscles touch, you stitch and choke for a while. Grab a tissue, wipe the eyes and blow the nose; next note!

Next note: five counts outward, hold; then five counts inward, hold. Move up the keyboard to as high as you can go. If you are unable to do both all the way up, then continue on with the one you are able to do, which will probably be your extones. Proceed up the keyboard as high as you can go, and then two notes higher. Then, bring it back down. Bring in the intones as soon as you can so as to be doing both extones and intones on each note for five counts. Go to as low as you can and then two notes lower.

Yes, this is difficult work. It is a work-out for your voice, but you must wake up your ligament. You may also find that your neck aches. These aches are due to the extrinsic tension dying out. (There were times when I would ache from my shoulders up to the top of my head.)

Rest a couple of minutes or so, maybe five. Now start as low as you can and extone all the way up for twelve counts, or as long as you are able if you cannot reach twelve. REMEMBER, TINY VOICE. You are working the very edge of your ligament. Relax! Now bring it all the way down, as low as you can, and then go two notes lower, attempting to sustain the sound for twelve counts.

Good Vibrations

What is your goal? This may seem impossible, but I assure you, it is not. Your goal is to have equal extone and intone sound for five octaves. To reach that takes time and work, and you may have an excellent voice and not need to go all the way, but that is the goal. Dr. Smolover claims this as a healthy ligament."

> "Most singers use only a small portion of their potential vocal range—usually about two octaves. However, to fully develop the voice and maximize its response in the singing range, the training range should extend from four to five octaves"[14]

My teacher had students whose voices were so high they went off the piano keyboard.

She would tell me, "Your progress will depend on many things, but one of the determining factors of your progress is just how weak your ligament is at the start. Some people may respond very quickly due to the fact that their voice is not all that bad. Others will take longer due to the poor condition of their voices.

Obviously, consistency of working the voice daily is an important factor. And remember that, as you work your voice, there will be changes that take place. As your voice begins to change, it may sound worse than when you started. Keep at it,

Third Workout, Third Month

and little by little, it will come in stronger. It will remain stronger for a while and then go weak. The change takes place again, and it comes back in stronger and better. This cycle happens over and over again."

At first I viewed the changes with fear and skepticism. Now I view them with excitement, knowing that when it comes back in it will be even better than before.

She would tell me, "Another thing you can expect is that, in one week, you may be able to reach certain notes and, in another week, you won't. Intones may work one week, and then may be hard to do the next, and vise versa. Do not panic. Keep working your voice, and little by little, it will come into new strengths and sounds, each time with a little stronger voice."

This is where my personal instructor was so helpful. She knew the ins and outs of the healing process. The duration of weeks for each exercise was guided by her experience. I was not to move to the next exercises too fast, especially because of my being spasmodic.

She would tell me trying to assure me everything would be alright, "It takes time to restore the voice, especially if you have SD. I know you want to talk, but be patient and do the work. You will be able to talk again."

Good Vibrations

SUMMARY OF WORKOUT:

I was to extone five counts; Intone five counts; up and down the keyboard. Do this first and once per work-out.

Extone twelve counts up, then two notes higher, and then down the keyboard, and two notes lower. Do this twice per work-out

Always end by going down the keyboard to your lowest note. Bring the ligament down.

I still hear her voice telling me these things, and in a way they are a fond memory, now that I am on this side of the trouble.

The following information seemed good, especially since it is in regards to spastic dysphonia:

"***Inspiratory phonation:*** Although it has been noted that patients with severe spastic dysphonia may resort to inspiratory phonation to get their massage across, instruction in the use of inspiratory phonation has only recently been reported in North America (Freeman and Shulman 1988). The successful use of this as a method for speaking in patients with spastic dysphonia, pioneered by Shulman (1989, personal communication), appears to offer an **effective approach to the management of some severely disabled pastients.** Shulman has also been experimenting with the use of inspiratory phonation as a relaxation technique for mild and moderately severe spastic dysphonic patients speaking on egressive air. Patients under her care report that **this is one of the most effective ways of relaxing laryngeal musculature.** Shulman has cautioned that inspiratory phonation must be done easily and with the throat open, otherwise the patient will experiance discomfort from the drying effect of the ingressive air stream."[11]

(Discomfort??? - Oh Yeah!!! You will choke. It is not easy at first. But it works and is worth it!)

Good Vibrations

9

4th Workout
Six Months

I was to continue six days a week with everything we had been doing, but now there were added a couple more exercises.

The exercise of extoning for five counts and then intoning for five counts was going to be cut down to three counts, and I was to try on each note not to pause very long. By that was meant, if I was at middle C, extone for three counts and then intone for three counts. I could take a breath between them, but try to not pause. Save the pause for when I moved to the next higher note. By doing this, I was flexing the ligament. This was always to be my first exercise. Go as high as I could, and then bring it down.

Good Vibrations

If I could not do both intones and extones all the way up, I was to go with the one that I could do as high as possible. When bringing my voice back down, I was to bring in both intones and extones as soon as I was able.

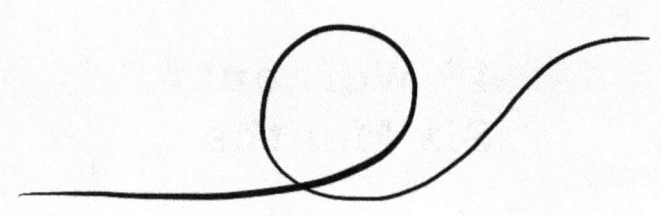

GLISSANDO: AKA Siren or sliding the voice

A Glissando is a smooth uninterrupted slide between pitches. This was to be my next exercise.
My teacher told me to:
"Start at the lowest note where you can make a clear sound and remember to work tiny. Start on this note and then slide your voice up one key. Then, without pausing, slide your voice back down to the original key. A total of two keys, for ½ step. On your piano, you will strike your first note and then strike the upper note, which would be one key higher. Then strike the lower note as you bring your voice down. Slide up one note, down one note, back up one note and back down one note, back up one note and back down one

4th Workout, Six Months

note, and hold for five counts.

Slide your voice up and then slide it back down all in one breath. It should take a total of about nine counts to do each time. Do your best. When you are sliding your voice, think of a circle. Do not stop at the upper note. Slide up to it and then slide back down and then slide back up and back down and hold for five counts. This is a mini glissando.

When you are ascending the keyboard on a mini glissando, start on the lower note and end on the lower note.

As you do the mini glissando descending from the top to the bottom, start on the higher note and end on the higher note when you are descending."

What was I doing to my ligament?

It was explained to me that as I "slid," with a clear tiny voice/sound, I was working the very edge of my ligament and, in a way, smoothing it out and increasing its ability to respond. Even though it is only two notes on the keyboard, it is like taking small steps up a steep mountain. Baby step by baby step I was working my way up and down my ligament. Slide up I was stetching it, and sliding down I was contracting it. The sliding was concentrating on the very edge as well.

I was to work my voice up the keyboard as high as I could go. There was no need to go two notes higher on this one. As my range would increase I was to bring it up farther in the future. Take a short rest, then bring it down.

At this point I was told to do the sustained intones and extones for 10 counts all the way up, and then all the way down the keyboard.

I was to always end descending and bringing my ligament down.

This was now a very extensive work-out. I was not to work my voice for more than an hour. That was too much. If I needed more time, I was to shorten my long sustained exercise to ten counts and do whole steps, or a scale.

I usually did every white note, but a scale cuts out some notes thus making the workout shorter.

SUMMARY OF MY WORKOUT

I was instructed to:

Alternate tones: Extone three counts, intone three counts, extone three, intone three, extone five. This was to be done on one breath with continuous sound. For a weak voice that is easier said than done!

Ascend to as high as you can, two notes higher, then descend to as low as you can, then two notes lower. Stretch on this exercise.

Mini Glissando: two-key range; slide voice up then down and back up and down; back up then down and hold 5 counts, tiny.

When ascending, start and end on lower note.
When descending, start and end on upper note.

Sustained Intone and Extone: Ten counts, ascending and descending the keyboard.

At this point, for SD, intoning is more important than extoning.

Good Vibrations

10

For The Very Weak Voice

When I started the Smolover method I had about eight notes on which I could make sound. Little by little, as the ligament strengthened and as I worked it, the range expanded to 10 notes, then 20, and now I have about five octaves on which I can make sound. But perhaps your voice is not as good as mine was. Maybe you are reading this and you have not spoken a word for some years.

As I started this book, I had not thought of that possibility until a lady contacted me who had not spoken above a whisper for five years. How would I even begin to work my voice if I did not have one? I thought about that for a while, and now offer a few thoughts for finding a starting place for my voice workouts.

I would sit at a piano or piano keyboard. I

Good Vibrations

would be hydrated, rested, and by myself in a distraction-free room. I like to pray and ask for the Lord Jesus Christ to help me.

After prayer, I would relax as best as i could and try to find somewhere on the keyboard where I could make a tiny sound. I have no idea where, as it would be different for a man or a woman as well as the person. I might try in the middle, or I might try up high. Maybe low, but I doubt it, because low sound takes strength and I had zero sound in my low end. I would find just one note where I could make a sound.

Remember, only ligament can make vibrational sound. Your voice is created when your ligaments come together (approximate) and vibrate as the air flows between them.

I would calmly search for just one note, however tiny the sound may be. I would try to relax and gently hum that note. That would be my ligament working. Hum some more, not louder but tiny, on the very edge. That would be my beginning. That one note would be the embryo I was going to develop for the growth of my voice. I would get used to coming to that note and humming. For the first two days I would just sit down and hum that note softly and tiny. The ebryo of my voice would grow from there. That would be home base, and I would build my voice from there.

I remember hearing of a man who was in the hospital after having a major operation. Many

For The Very Weak Voice

people did not recover from the condition he had, but after lying in bed for a few days, he determined tomorrow he was going to sit up. It was not easy and took great effort, but the next day he did sit up. The next day after that he decided he was going to sit on the edge of his bed for a certain length of time, and he did. He then decided he was going to stand on his feet the next day, and he did. The next day he took a step, and the next day more and more.

I had eight notes, but even if I would of had only one weak note where I could make sound, that would be my starting point. I would have to find that one place where I could make sound. From there, I would build my voice.

If I couldn't make sound by extones (i.e. air flowing out of the lungs), which is the normal method, then I would have to try pulling air into my lungs and making sound that way. Intones have been proven to be extremely helpful for those afflicted with SD.

One way or another, I would find that first note, that first sound. And when I did, I would need to realize that right there my ligament was working. Right there it was coming together and vibrating. Right there would be my foundation, and from there, I would begin to rebuild my voice.

I would remind myself that it is going to take time, so I must be very patient.

If I found that place where I could make sound

Good Vibrations

then I would hum a tiny sound there. How long? As long as I wanted, and just listen to myself making sound.

The next day, I would hum again and, this time, try the next note higher. I would be gentle. Hum my good note, and then strike the next key and try to hum the next higher note. If that does not work, try the next note lower. Softly and gently, if possible.

Then I would return to my first note, or "home base," and try sliding my voice up into the next note and then hold it there briefly. Try that again. Home base hum and then try sliding up to the next note, and then slide back down to home base. This sliding upward or downward between two notes is called a glissando, and it would be my beginning.

I would do this for a couple of days; three or four times in one day. Just do those two notes. Try to get to where I could do the two notes without having to slide my voice. Extone on the first note and then extone on the second note.

On the third or fourth day, hum extone at home base for three counts if I could. Hum the next higher note for three counts if I could.

Now slide my voice from home base to the next higher note and back down. I would do this twice. Then I would start at the note just above home base and try to slide to the next higher note. If it doesn't work, I would rest a bit. Come back later

For The Very Weak Voice

that day and try again.

The next day I would start at home base and hum tiny for three counts. Hum the next higher note for three counts. If I was not able to, then I would try sliding up to it. I would try to slide my voice up to it and then back down to home base. Then I would try humming on the second note up from home base. If I could hum on it, then I would try sliding it up one note higher. Softly and gently, relax and slide up to the next note and, without stopping, slide back down to the lower note.

If I was only able to make sound by humming inward, then I would do this exercise by humming inward. Once I could make sound by humming inward, then I would try to hum outward on the same note. Softly and gently, I would hum a tiny sound inward. Stop, breathe, and try to hum outward, seeing if I could make just a tiny sound. I would listen for it, and then I would build upon it, ever mindful that it would take persistance and great patience.

If intones are easier, I would stay with them for a while. Hum on my home base. Then try to hum one note higher. Hum on my home base and slide my voice up into the next note with my intones, and then try to slide my voice back down.

It might seem so small, yet when I would be done, I would feel a bit tired. This is work! I would be concentrating, as well as working a part of my body that has not worked for a while. I need to take my time. Don't get impatient. Note by note, my voice will grow.

Once I would have brought in the next note up, I would keep trying for the next one higher, then higher. Slide my voice into the next one higher, and then slide it back down. If I had two notes that worked well, then I would try the mini glissando on them and work them. I would try doing extones for three counts, then a few days later, for five counts, and a few days later for seven counts. Little by little I would solidify what voice I had.

At this point, it would not translate into speaking sound, but in time, it will. As the ligament expands in its ability and response, little by little I would find that I was beginning to be able to speak. Still I would have to remind myself not to get in a hurry. It takes time, but I would know that I was making progress and that I was on the path of voice restoration.

Examples of Glissandos used in various therapies:

Glide from your lowest to your highest note on the word "knoll" or on a lip or tongue trill. Voice should be soft, and a forward focus used. If breaks occur, continue to glide without hesitating.[4]

"...glide downward...then glissando back to the 'little oo' on the high note. Again, go up by half steps as far as is comfortable according to the nature of the voice. The voice cannot resonate a sound which is not in the glottal source."[15]

Vocal Function Exercises

There are four steps to the program: (a) vocal warm-up by sustaining the vowel "ee" for as long as possible, (b) stretching of the laryngeal muscles by **gliding** from the lowest note to the highest note, (c) contracting of the laryngeal muscles by **gliding** from the highest note to the lowest note, and (d) building muscular power by sustaining musical notes for as long as possible... The exercises are to be done softly without excess strain.[16]

Good Vibrations

11

5th Workout
One Year

It is hard to remember exactly when each of these exercises were incorporated into my workout. With each person I am sure there are variables of how long it takes to bring in new exercises. The important thing for me was stressed that I was to work out six days a week for an hour or less. Because I was working with ligaments and muscles it is very much the same as going to a gym. But with the voice it is daily. Many of the new vocal function exercises developed by places like John's Hopkins and Greater Baltimore Medical Center recommend the exercises be done twice a day though the work out is much shorter.

From now on, each work-out session was to start with this exercise.

THE NEW WARM-UP:

Start as low as possible on the keyboard. Relax and think tiny and clear! Deep breath, breath out some and now tiny extone for two counts, intone for two counts, extone for two counts, intone for two counts, extone and hold for five counts, if you can. That was my goal. Go up the keyboard as high as I could go. I did not have to bring it down; just ascend to the highest note that I was able. If, in the beginning, I could not make sound on both ex-tone and intone, then I was to go as high as I could on both. Then if extones are the only ones working, go as high as I could on them and try for two notes higher. If it is intones only, then go with them. STRETCH!

REGULAR GLISSANDO:

Now instead of the mini glissando, I was instructed to do a regular glissando. I was going to span five notes for this exercise and would only circle up and down twice. From my starting note, not fast not slow, slide up four notes and down to the starting note, then up four notes and down to the starting note, up four notes and hold for five counts, if possible. Alternate starting note from extone to intone all the way up the keyboard.

Glissandos are done in one breath. Do not stop

Fith Workout, One Year

and take a breath in the middle of a glissando. If it is extone, I took a deep breath before starting. If I was intoning, then I was to empty my lungs before starting the glissando. Glissando's are done in one breath. It is also a good work-out for the lungs.

Start at the same note as I did for the warm-up exercise. Ascend up the keyboard, alternating on each starting note. By that I was to extone glissando on a note. The next note up I was to do the same thing intoning. Do this all the way up the keyboard to as high as I could. There was no need to go two notes higher.

Glissando's work the flex, the stretch, and making the ligament responsive with the slide. It is a way of patching up the "holes" on the edge of the ligament.

Those two exercises now made up my warm-up routine. I was to always start with these two exercises. They are the foundation of my work-out.

These get the ligament ready for the work-out. I would generally work my voice for an hour. I had to realize though, that when working the voice up high, it greatly fatigues the ligament. There would be times when I would skip a day so my ligament could rest. They told me six days a week, but sometimes my instructor would tell me on Tuesday to not work it until seeing her again at my next session on Thursday, giving the

Good Vibrations

ligament a one day rest. This was usually requested when she wanted a rested ligament to test and determine its progress. Again, this is where an instructor is helpful. I would push myself, but there would be times when I would pause a day and let my ligament rest. It was just one of those things that I had to experiment with to see what worked best for me.

Intones: Start at the top, on my highest note. Think tiny, tiny, way up high, seemingly up behind the nose. It is work, but I was to reach for the very highest where I could make a tiny sound. Even if it was only for two or three counts, start there. This was ligament only (Modality One) sound. Now bring it down, attempting to go ten counts with intone only. Intones bypass extrinsic tension, therefore they are very good for the ligament. Bring this down as low as I could on the keyboard.

What I was doing is bringing Modality One, or ligament only, down as low as I could. Since only ligament makes sound and, when it is strong, it can work without help, this exercise helps strengthen it. As it is able to come down, the vocal ability will goes up.

Rest for a few minutes.

Now, I was to do a mini glissando exercise. Start low and ascend the keyboard to the top. Start on the low note and end on the low note.

Fifth Workout, One Year

From the top, do a mini glissando, bringing it down. When descending, start the mini glissando on the upper note and finish on the upper note.

Now I was going to do a cool-down. The cool-down is always done by descending. I was instructed to always finish the workout by descending because it brings the ligament down. Little by little, it will respond.

Start as high as possible. Sometimes it would be about three notes lower than at the start because my ligament was tired. Extone for two counts, then intone for two counts, then extone for two counts. Move down to the next note, starting with intone on the note, extone, then intone. Move down to next note and start with extone, then intone, and so on, always alternating the extone and intone. Bring it down to as low as possible.

That is the end of this work out.

Whether it was a year or a year and a half before I got to this point I'm not sure, but from here on this was the standard workout for a while. Month after month I was to work on perfecting each exercise. Remember to think tiny and clear. Relax and be consistent to work my voice six days a week.

If my voice sounded worse, I was to keep working through it, six days a week, and when it came back in, it was a little better. I was told over and over, "Do not panic." This is part of the rebuilding. Remember, I was dealing with ligament so it would take time.

SUMMARY OF WORKOUT:

1. **Warm up alternating ascending:** two out, two in, two out, two in, five out.
2. **Regular Glissando alternating ascending:** 5-note range - slide up four notes, then down, then up four notes then down, then up four and hold for 5 counts. The next note up, alternate to intone, then next note higher extone.
    A. Still today at the writing of this book my first octave is the regular Glissando on extones only because I have no intone down low.
3. **Intone sustained ten counts descending:** start at top
4. **Mini glissando:** ascend and descend the keyboard
5. **Cool-down, descending only:** start at top

12

Two Year Mark

By this time there was noticeable improvement in my voice. Though it was still poor. But it showed that my voice was headed in the right direction. I had experienced a few vocal changes where my voice initially seemed "out of control" and then emerged a little bit better and stronger.

I was now able to differentiate between my ligament only, which is Modality One, and ligament with muscle, which is Modality Two. My voice was very poor at the start, and I was not able to properly discern Modality Three. It was only discernable in the lower register and for girls, it is a bit harder to distinguish. Females rarely use Modality Three, though it is a part of the "vocal team" used in the production of sound.

Good Vibrations

I now also had hope. I was able to see that my voice was not broken or "terminal", but that it could be rehabilitated. Hope is a good thing.

I know what it is like to come into an office in tears thinking I may never communicate again with words. I know what it is like to consider having to do sign language as if I were clinically dumb (not being able to speak and make sound). So many fearful thoughts ran through my mind when my voice did not work properly.

So now, I am going to bring in some different exercises. They basically do what I had already been doing, but were a bit more specific. Again, This is one of those places where my personal instructor was helpful. A personal instructor merely speeds up the rehabilitation. But I think many people are more than capable of rehabilitating their own voice by doing these exercises consistently and properly.

I know one thing for sure. If my voice had been healthy when I started these exercises, it would have responded very quickly with tonal improvement as well as expansion of my range for singing. There would have been the changes to go through, but coming out the other side would be great.

I remember reading a review of Raymond Smolover's *Sing Your Best* which is the method that was used on me to restore my voice. One of the reviews gave the book only one star because the reviewer said that he lost his voice when he did the exercises. He had no idea that what he was going through was normal and would come out better on the other side. Dr. Smolover never mentioned this in the book.

A REMINDER:

I had been working my voice for five years, with the last two of those being on my own. I had some extra money left for a lesson and I was not far from where my instructor lived so I scheduled a voice work-out.
It was so good to see her and sit in the chair that I had sat in for three years, twice a week. Memories flooded my mind of those times.
After our greeting and prayer, she reached out and pressed the piano key and said, "Warm up." I began to hum extone and immediately she said, "Softly, tiny." I backed off and realized I had been doing them too loudly.
So remember to work "tiny" with the clearest, softest sound. This will enable you to work the very edge of your ligament, for that is where sound is created by the vibrations of the ligament. In the tiny is your strength.

Good Vibrations

I WAS GIVEN A NEW WORK OUT:

Warm up as usual alternating extones and intones all the way up the keyboard.

I was to do the Regular Glissando, alternating all the way up. And I was able to sustain longer, so I was intructed to do two circles of the regular glissando and then hold the last note for five counts if I could. (In Dr. Smolover's book, *Sing Your Best*, he has the student doing three circles and then the holding.)

I was to start at the lowest notes where I could make sound. A female should attempt -C2, which is two octaves below middle C. Males should now be starting at -C3, which is three octaves below middle C, even if you have no sound. For the first octave I was only able to do extones, so that is what I did.

Then I was to start my alternating of tones as soon as I was able which was about an octave higher from where I started.

She again told me that if my voice was not perfect don't worry about it. If I was at a gym and given new exercises, it would be a while before you could do them perfectly. I was not to be distracted by what I perceived as imperfection. I was to just do the exercises and, in time, it will all come together.

STALLED OR MOVING?

As I began working my voice, it would take "extra" time to do each exercise. When I would move to the next note, it would take time to work it there. At the beginning of rehab my voice ligament was be very stiff and inoperable in places. The whole purpose of this therapy was to reverse that and to get my ligament strong, flexible and functional. So I would stall a bit at each note for the first few months. It was understandable, but now I am to keep my progression up the keyboard moving. There is a balance to this, but I am instructed not to get sidetracked by over analyzing the sound I am making.

My goal is tiny and clear, which is much easier now. Tiny is important and necessary, but clear has developed the more and longer I do the exercises. I am to try to keep moving to the next note. This will help remove the extrinsic tension. Making sound has to become as involuntary as it was before my voice problems began. There was a time when I did not even think about how to make sound; it was just there, and I could talk. Restoration of this ability is one of my goals, so I am to try to keep moving, and to stay relaxed, as well.

There is a fine line between "relax" and "keep moving." To move can cause me to tense, but to

Good Vibrations

be slow can cause me to bring in extrinsic tension. I am not to be overwhelmed by these facts. My voice will come through if I keep working it. These are just some reminders to be aware of as I work my voice, especially now that I am at (and beyond) the one-year mark. In the beginning, there was no way for me to understand what I am talking about here and even less ability to put it into practice.

There were times when I would go for my lesson and my instructor would move me and not let me slow down. The tiny, clear sound would be "all messed up," and I would think that I had done a horrible job that day. At the end of the lesson she would say, "Good work out. You did a good job today," and I could tell she was not just trying to make me feel good. She heard things that I did not hear. So, if I keep it moving and it doesn't sound perfect, I am not to let that trouble me. Keep it moving, keep it tiny and keep working my voice. Little by little, it will return, and it has.

Ok, I have done my two warm ups.

The next exercise has been a great help for spasmodics, at least according to my instructor. It is a small glissando, also known as, what I call the mini glissando.

I start at my lowest note (-C2 for ladies and -C3 for men). I slide up one key, a half-step, and then back down to the starting note. Slide up one, down one, up one, down one, up one, down one,

Two Year Mark

and end on the down, or original, note. This will be done with extones. Relax, tiny, extone, slide up one note, then down three times, ending on the low note and holding for five counts.

   I do this all the way up, to as high as I am able, and then bring it down. By now, females should be approaching +C3, and males you should be approaching +C2. I do not always make it to these goals, but that is where I am aiming. At times my voice will do better than at other times. At times I am able to go higher than other times, and the same is true for going lower. Oh how I remember my instructor saying, "Just keep working it, and you will be fine." She would tell me this over and over, and she was right.

   One other note that I would like to make here is that I cannot go too high. Actually the higher the better, but only as the ligament is able.

   I am to do this mini glissando up, and then do it all the way down, but when I descend, I am to finish on the high note. I am to start my descending mini glissando on the upper note and finish on the upper note. So, going up the keyboard, I will start on the lower note and finish on the lower note. Going down the keyboard, I will start on the upper note and finish on the upper note.

   My workout now is to do this exercise, the mini glissando, up and down the keyboard twice. Remember to slide my voice. Don't stop at the top or bottom note; slide my voice. I am working the very edge of my voice, inching it up and down; smoothing it out for a better response. This is a very important exercise.

At times I do some long sustained intones or extones, for about twelve counts. If I choose one over the other, I choose intones for SD, and finish them descending.

At this point it is time to do the cool down exercise descending, and keep it moving. Don't wait for it. Also, on my cool down, work the voice small, and when I am up high, it will seem like it is right behind my nose. Work with small, relaxed movement. This will free me up to be able to move better. Sounds up high may be rough, just keep it moving and bring it down.

There are many times that I still stich and choke. It just means I have more work to do. When I stitch or choke, it shows that I am working my voice and trying to expand its ability to stretch and flex. Good job! Keep at it. It also means that my ligament is still weak and is collapsing to the point where the muscles are touching, thus creating the sensation that causes me to "stitch". Some days I do not want to choke so I may work my voice a bit easier. That is all right and is normal. But there will be times, where I need to challenge and push my ligament for a good work out.

It is no different than lifting weights or working

Two Year Mark

out at the gym. Some days you take it easy, and other days you push yourself. I need to try to keep the effort on to improve my voice. You will be so glad you did, though it is hard work. I must not forget that! This is work that very few will be able to understand. I must walk this road in order to understand this road.

This workout now is going to be my core workout. It flexes, strengthens and aligns the ligament. Consistent daily working, five to six days a week, will bring my voice in. Week after week, and I have sensed great improvement, or I should say hear, improvement. My ligament is responding little by little, and it is exciting!

My instructor told me it would take five years for my voice to be completely corrected. I had to quit the lessons after three years, for financial reasons, but I have absolutely no doubt that if I had been able to stay and do the lessons for two more years, my voice would be better than it had ever been in my life.

With the Smolover method, I am working my voice, which consists of muscles and ligaments. Therefore, with proper continued working of my voice, it will continue to improve to a point where it is the best it has ever been in my whole life.

If you consistently exercise your body, does it not get better and better? You are working the muscles and ligaments of your body. It is no different with the muscles and ligaments of the

Good Vibrations

voice, for my voice operates through the sound of the ligaments and the teamwork of the muscles surrounding it. If I get all those parts in shape and working right, I will have an excellent voice. This is the basis of the Smolover method.

It is now over 50 years since Dr. Smolover set out to find a way to get the voice back. The wonder of the Smolover method is its simplicity. Well, mental simplicity. If your voice is weak, it is work.

SUMMARY OF WORKOUT:

I was indtructed not to go over 60 minutes.

1. **Warm-up, alternating ascending**: two out, two in, two out, two in, five out.
2. **Regular Glissando, alternating ascending**: slide up four notes, then down, then up, then down, then up and hold for five, next note intone. Covers a total of five notes.
3. **Optional**: Extone sustained ten counts descending.
4. **Intone sustained ten counts descending**: Best for SD.
5. **Mini Glissando**: three circles: 1/2 step, next white key higher - slide up one, down one, three times and hold for five counts if you can. Do this all on one breath if you can. Don't take a breath to finish; it is what it is. In time, it will hold. Do

this up and down the keyboard.

6. **Cool-down, descending:** Two out, two in, two out – keep it moving down the keyboard. Don't stall; just keep moving, regardless of what it sounds like. Use tiny movement right up behind the nose.

Anatomic/Physiologic Explanation

Practice on maximal prolongations should improve strength and endurance of vocal fold muscles and the coordination of respiration and phonation. By performing pitch glides to high and low pitches, the cricothyroid and vocal fold muscles should be lengthened and shortened, inducing flexibility and strength.[16]

Dr. Jackie Gartner-Schmidt

Good Vibrations

13

Extra Exercises

Now and then I try these and see how I do with them. A work-out should be no longer than 60 minutes. I nearly always do the mini glissando. It has been a help to me, but only after a few months of doing it with the extones only.

I try these other exercises, but in order to tell if they are helping, I need to incorporate them into my workout consistently for a month before I can tell what effect they are having.

The only exercise that could cause harm is the crescendo on the ligament, if I do it incorrectly. (The harm is that it will produce extrinsic tension. It will not damage the ligament.) There is nothing to worry about with the other exercises.

At the beginning of my lessons, there were some

Good Vibrations

exercises that my instructor would occasionally have me do. About a year and a half into my work, Dr. Smolover retired. My instructor would still consult with him from time to time, but she was on her own and quite capable, at that.

Every now and then, she would tweak things a bit. As I was able to get back to preaching, I would be away from her instruction for months at a time. Sometimes I would schedule a phone work-out with her, and it would be a great help to me, but there was nothing like being there in person with her. More than once I would come in, and by the end of the lesson, my voice was fantastic. She knew just what to do and how.

So here are some other exercises that, from time to time I try. They are variations of what I am already doing.

When I first began to work my voice, all I was concerned with was making sound. It didn't matter how, though I was to try to keep it tiny. Yet in the beginning, even that was not possible. I was just trying to make sound any way I could.

This was to be expected, especially because my ligament was severely collapsed. Then my ligament began to "wake up" and respond; it started to "come in," so to speak. As I would ascend the keyboard, or note scale, I noticed at certain points along the way my voice changed, and the way I made sound changed.

My voice went from breathy to clearer, and so

Extra Exercises

on. After some months, I was able to determine what is ligament only. The ligament will only work on its own on intones, which is why intones are so important in isolating the ligament. But the ligament will also work on its own with extones when it is in shape. It is in the upper register where ligament-only works. The goal is to bring it down and to strengthen it.

LIGAMENT CRESCENDO:

I was told that this exercise is to be performed on ligament only, known as Modality One. If a person does not know for sure if it is modality one, then they should not do this exercise. This exercise is to strengthen the dynamic range of the ligament. I would say this is more for singers who have a healthy vocal instrument.

I am to start at my highest note and sustain the extone. Then on the second or third count, use more force. In a way I am bearing down on the ligament. My sound will become louder. Hold for one count and then back off to a soft, tiny sound.

If I bring in Modality Two, which is muscle, I will defeat the exercise. This exercise is to be done on Modality One (ligament only), and I must have a semi-strong ligament to begin with in order to accomplish this exercise.

Good Vibrations

MINI GLISSANDO:

I am going to again stress that I have had great success with this exercise, performed by extones, for Spasmodic Dysphonia. Remember to do it tiny, and you can perform it by alternating the tones or by intone only, as well as extone only, as I have already described.

In other words, the mini glissando is good for the voice whether intoning, extoning, or alternating between the two.

LARGE GLISSANDO:

A large glissando is one that my instructor would have me do at times. Instead of covering only five keys, the large glissando covers a span of seven keys. This obviously works a larger portion of the ligament all at once, over and over, as you move up and down the keyboard. It is to be done the same way as the other glissandos, only slide the voice up seven keys and then down to the beginning key.

Get a lot of air for this one on extones, and empty the lungs for intones. This one exercise will need sustained tone for 10-14 counts.

NEW SOUNDS:

After consistently doing these exercises, I began to hear sounds that I had never heard my ligament make before. They would usually occur when I was way up high. They will be very tiny and would come in from above, or over the top. At first they would just happen, and I would have no control over them. I was instructed to try to "catch" it and bring it in. As I continued to work my ligament, I would bring this sound in and then bring it down. With each new sound, I would gain freedom, range, and strength in my voice.

SUMMARY OF WORKOUT:

I was to always end the work-out session by bringing my voice down, descending.

Glissando illustration - Done with one, two, or three loops of the voice and then sustained.

Good Vibrations

14

The Exercises Illustrated

For audio examples of the exercises go to http://spasmodicdysphoniavoice.com

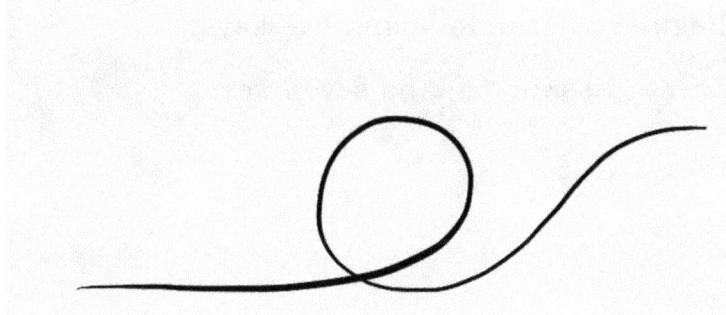

Glissando - a sliding of the voice

Good Vibrations

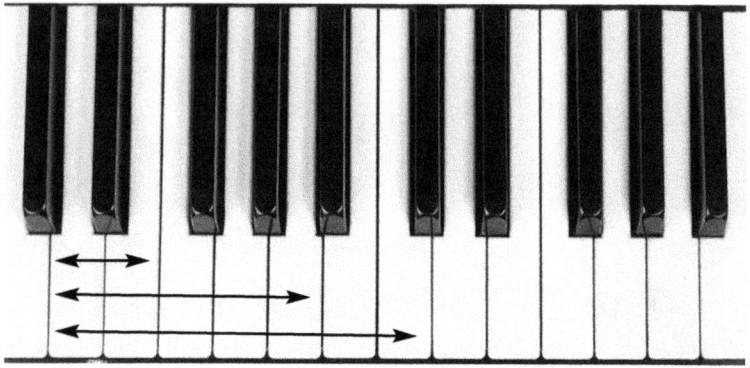

1. Mini glissando spans two keys.
2. Regular glissando spans five keys.
3. Large glissando spans seven keys.

The Exercises Illustrated

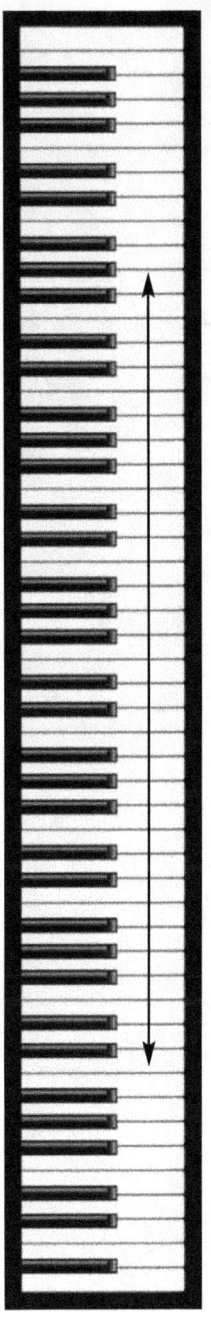

1. Extones - 5 counts:

Introductory exercise – works the stretch. In the beginning I was to make sound any way I could. I was only to be able to make sound for an octave, but worked up to five octaves. I was to bring it to a tiny clear sound when I could.

She told me to, "Move up as high as you can and then down the keyboard to as low as you can."

Good Vibrations

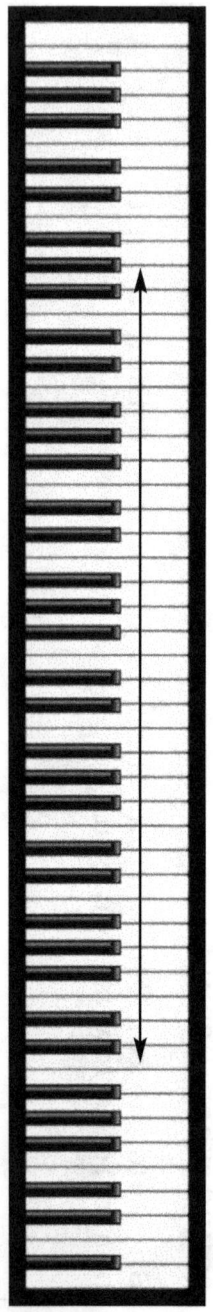

2. Extones - 12 counts:

Introductory exercise – Works the stretch and builds strength. At times I held the extones for twenty counts. She told me to move up as high as I could and then down the keyboard to as low as I was able.

The Exercises Illustrated

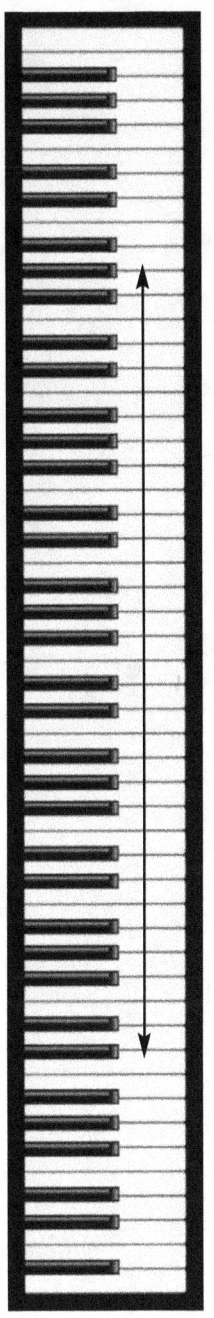

3. Extone 5 counts then Intone 5 counts:

Intermediate exercise to work the flex of the ligament as well as preparing you for your warm up exercise.

She told me to start at your lowest note and hum out five counts, then with little to no break hum inward for five counts. Ascend to your highest note and then descend to your lowest note.

Good Vibrations

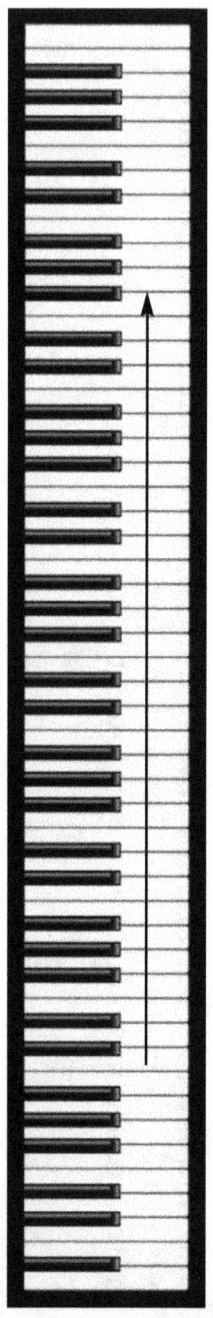

4. Standard warm-up exercise:

Smooth intone then extone – extone 2 counts then intone 2 counts, extone 2 counts, intone 2 counts then extone and hold 5 counts. This works your flex and stretch as well as warming you up for your work out.

Only ascend on this work out. No need to bring it down.

The Exercises Illustrated

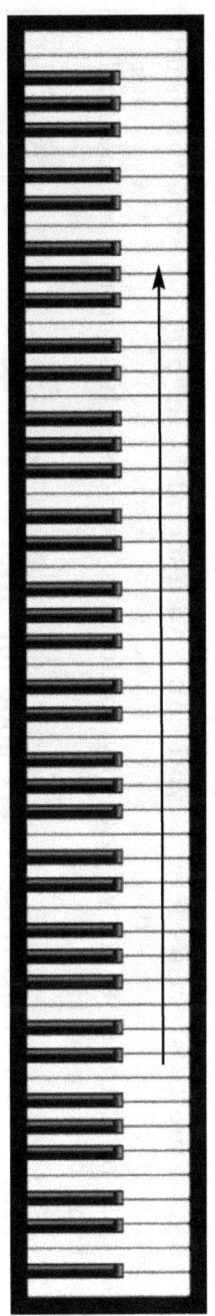

5. Warm-Up Glissando:

She told me to alternate as you ascend - All in one breath, slide up 5 keys and slide back down to first note then slide up to top key and hold it for 5 counts. Start as low as you can and ascend to as high as you can. Slide your voice not too fast, but not slow either.

Intermediate yet standard exercise - works response, flex, stretch, and smooths out the ligament edge.

Good Vibrations

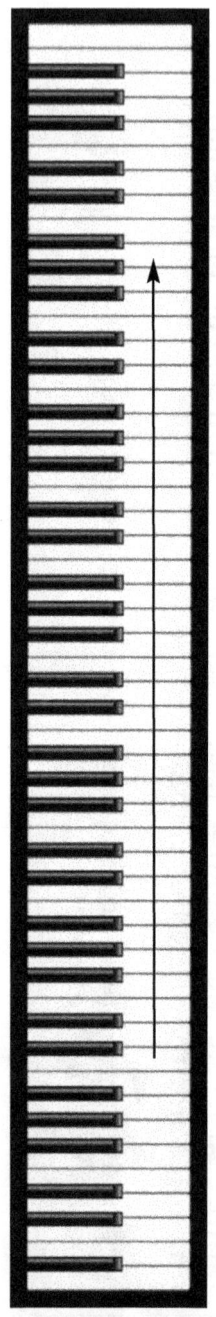

6. Sustained Intones:

Intone for ten to twenty counts. The muscles of Modalities Two and Three cannot help the ligament. The ligament has to work on it's own, thus freeing it up from extrinsic tension which is extremely important.

She told me to start as low as you can and ascend to as high as you can, and then bring it back down to as low as you can. Make sound any way you can on this one; there is no wrong way to do this exercise, just make sound and in time clear and tiny.

General work out exercise – very good for SD.

The Exercises Illustrated

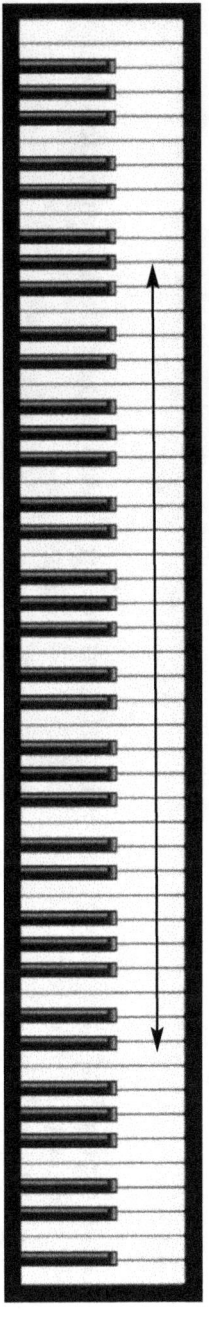

7. Mini-Glissando:

3 circles – mostly done extone only but can be intone or alternate. Slide up one key, 1/2 step, and back down, up, down, up, down and hold 5 counts. Ascending - start low and end low. Descending - start upper key and end upper key.

Strength, response, and stretch.

Very good and essential exercise for SD students as well as anyone.

Good Vibrations

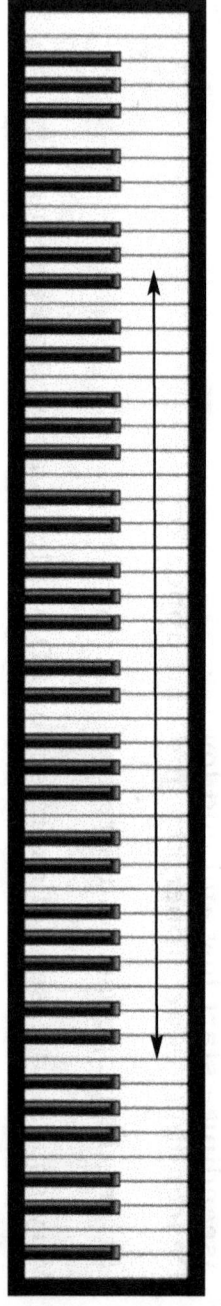

8. Regular Glissando:

Two to three "circles" of the voice then bring up to high note and hold for five counts. You will need a lot of breath for this exercise. If your breath just passes through do your best and in time you will be able to do this one.

9. Large Glissando:

One "circle" of the voice but you will move up seven notes then back down to low note and hold for three counts.

Both of these are performed to as high as you can and then down to as low as you can.

The Exercises Illustrated

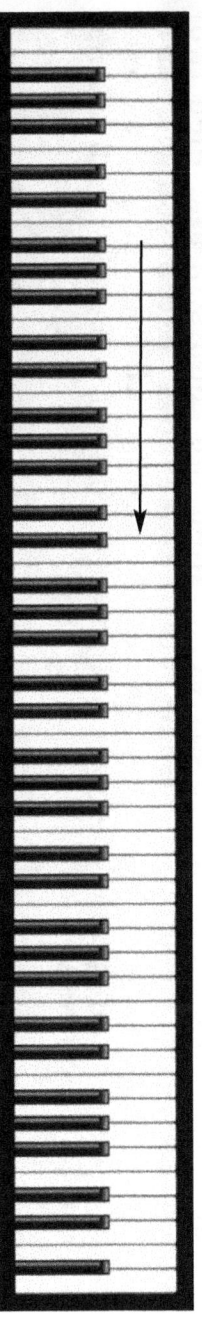

10. Ligament Crescendo - this is a technical exercise:

Ligament only - extone sustain 2 counts, crescendo on ligament only 2 counts, diminuendo (Diminish) for 2 counts – total of 6 counts for this exercise.

Do not bring muscle in or this exercise build extrinsic tension. If you perform this exercise correctly you will not be able to bring it all the way down. Only work it where you know you are on ligament only. If you cannot discern if you are working ligament only do not do this exercise.

Builds dynamic range of ligament.

Good Vibrations

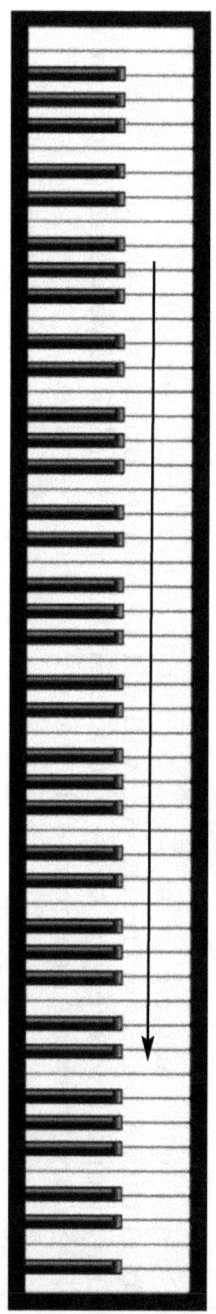

11. Cool Down:

She told me that at the end of your work out you are to do the cool down. This is very important for bringing the new behavior in by bringing the ligament down. Start up as high as you are able. Hum two counts in and then two counts out, then two counts in. Same thing next key lower except you will start with extone two counts, intone two counts and extone two counts. Each starting note will be opposite of the previous one. Keep your voice moving bringing it down to as low as you can.

The Exercises Illustrated

Some of the exercises will help the muscles and ligament work together, but the most important modality to work is Modality One, the ligament. If I do nothing else, I must free it up from extrinsic tension, strengthen it, align it, and flex it so it can stand on its own. Modality One is where the voice is born.

For SD, intones are very important in strengthening and freeing up the ligament. Ligament cannot use muscle to make sound on intones.

One last thing that I must remember: It will take time, depending on the condition of my ligament at the start and how quickly it responds to the exercises. Take your time, step by step, day by day five to six days a week. Work your voice and, unless your ligament is physically damaged, you can have your voice back. You will talk again!

As of this writing I am talking again and singing with my guitar as well. I never dreamed that I would do that again!

Good Vibrations

15

A Glimpse Of The Path

Over the past few years, I have had a few people who have been diagnosed with SD contact me and ask for help. Subsequently, I have instructed them on how to work their voices, step by step, so as to recover from SD. The writing of this book is an attempt to give my tesatimony to others that they might be able to do the same without having to contact me or anyone else. Though, as I have already stated, the best way is to have a personal instructor to guide you in your voice recovery.

My desire in adding this chapter is to give you a time frame, as well as a working example, of those who have, and are, performing these exercises. This may answer or shed some light on the work-out in a way that I have not been able to do in the mere description of the work-out. What you will

Good Vibrations

see is the work-out and progress in action, as well as the fears, questions and joys from those who have traveled this path. As my instructor told me, "You have to travel the path in order to teach it." So I have traveled this path, and here are a few more that are traveling the path as of the writing of this book.

As Connie Pike has mentioned in her book, it is a comfort to read and hear of others who have SD and to hear of their struggles as you can relate to them. There are so few who understand your frustrations, depression and despair, at times.

For the purpose of privacy, I have changed the names of these people. The first person I will call "Windy", and the second, I will call "Breezy".

FIRST CONTACT:

Oct 12, 2012
Windy wrote:
Dear Pastor McDonald,
I wrote an email to your church website and then found this email address this evening when I read your testimony again. It is truly inspirational to me and gives me great hope. I, too, after several bouts with bronchitis was diagnosed with ABSD about four and a half years ago...almost five. My voice deteriorated very slowly over a period of about a year. I am a kindergarten teacher and noticed that my voice

was slowly breaking and becoming breathy and weak over several months. I spent two years at various doctors and was diagnosed with ABSD about two years or so ago. I did have thyroid surgery as well and my laryngeal nerve was tethered around a large nodule that the doctors removed. They are not sure whether though this contributed or not to my SD. I attended Connie Pikes clinic in Florida this past March and have made some progress but my voice is still so weak and breathy....I am whispering most of the time. I have taken a leave of absence from my job.

I have read your story and if you could help in any way with directing me to A. R. and her method of voice therapy, I would so appreciate it. I did have two Botox injections early on but the side effects were so debilitating. I aspirated eight times in two months and had breathing problems. I decided that they were out of the question for me. I am willing to try anything!! My faith is strong and that does sustain me in this journey. I feel very blessed yet I do want to keep persevering with voice therapy, it seems to be the only option with ABSD.

If you would be so kind to direct me with how I can reach A. V. and possibly begin voice therapy I would so appreciate it. I live in Virginia but maybe she could help me via skype or give me exercises to work on.

Thank-you so much,
Windy

Good Vibrations

Oct 13, 2012
Dear Windy,

I understand your frustration with ABSD! Forgive me for not getting back to you sooner. Here is A. daughter's email address as she is a contact person to get in contact with A. A. is about 90 years old and just had an operation for breast cancer. She is still working with people though and has another lady who only works with Spasmodics.

I remember A. telling me that she had a student, a middle aged woman, who had asthma. As something to do she came to A. for voice lessons for singing. After a few years of doing this therapy her asthma was gone. I will say when I was doing the therapy it did strengthen my lungs and increased their capacity.

Hope this helps. God bless,
Ken McDonald

June 19, 2013
Dear Windy,

I just came across your email again. I had forgotten about it. How are you doing with you ABSD? I have worked with some people by email and they have been helped. I just saw your email and am wondering if you have been helped yet.

I am in the process of writing a book on the

exercises as to how to get your voice back, but it will be a while before it is published.
Sincerely
Ken McDonald

June 19, 2013,
Dear Ken,
Hello! Thank-you so very much for emailing me! I am doing a little better with my ABSD but after five years not nearly where I would like to be. I meet with a singing coach twice a month...we are trying different things but my progress has been slow! I did attend Connie Pikes clinic over a year ago and her exercises helped too yet not enough to sustain my voice over time. My voice is still breathy and weak a lot of the time. Most of the time all I can do is whisper. I would love your help if you would be so kind to email me with the exercises that worked over time for you....I am so very grateful for your email! I thought that you may just have been so busy that you could not respond....thank-you so much.
Looking forward to hearing from you,
Windy

(This is the start of her working her voice.)

June 19, 2013
Dear Windy,
I am so glad you wrote back. I would be glad to

Good Vibrations

help you. I am writing a book on how I got my voice back from SD with the exercises in it so that others can get their voices restored. I have worked with some people and they have had excellent results.

There is so much I could write, but I will give you what you need to start. The book will explain it all so much better.

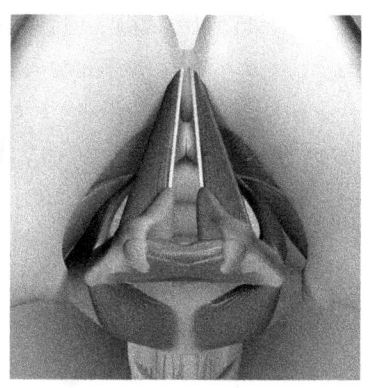

I went on Google and put in vocalis muscle, images. You will notice on this image the vocal ligament. That is what makes vibrational sound. The reason your voice is breathy is because your ligament is not approximating correctly, which means it is not coming together so that when the air passes between it does not vibrate. What you need is for your ligament to approximate.

My voice did the same thing.

Next to the ligament you have the vocalis muscle and then the thyroarytenoid muscle. It is with these three "modalities" that a larynx makes

A Glimpse of The Path

sound. So your voice is produced by ligaments and muscles and just as you can pull a muscle or ligament, or you get out of shape, so too these muscles and ligaments can get faulty, or out of shape and need to be brought back into condition where they have Strength, alignment and flex. But remember that only the ligament makes sound. Muscle cannot make sound, so it is imperative that your ligament gets restored.

What you need:

A piano or a piano keyboard

A place where you can be undistracted while you do your exercises

Though not absolutely important but when you do your exercises be hydrated, do not be dehydrated.

Here is your first exercise with an explanation of what you are doing and why.

These exercises are going to be work so prepare yourself.

You are going to stretch your ligament in order to get it limber. It is a basic exercise but is the beginning of getting your voice back.

You are seated upright at your piano or keyboard with no phone and will be uninterrupted. You will need to concentrate on what you are doing. This won't be hard for the first few months.

Good Vibrations

Relax. I pray before starting.

At the start you will just have to experiment on where you will start but middle C generally is a good place.

Find about where the lowest note you are able to make tiny clear sound at. At the first any sound will do.

VERY IMPORTANT: You are to hum with your mouth closed, and the sound is to be your tiny and clear. Only sound is made from your ligament, and you want to work the very edge of your ligament. Very tiny and clear if you are able.

Start at the lowest note and hum outward extone for 5 counts or seconds. You are very relaxed and concentrating. Now go to the next note higher. With each note higher you are going to stretch your ligament. The higher you go your ligament thins out and stretches.

Go to as high as you are able on the keyboard. Once you have reached as high as you can go, try to go two notes higher. S-T-R-E-T-C-H. It is work! Take a short break, then start at the top and hum out for 5 counts and bring it all the way down to as low as you can go. When you get as low as you can, try to go two notes lower.

Do this exercise three times, or for 30-40 minutes once a day, six days a week. This is your beginning workout.

Relax and make sound anyway you can and

then try to back off and make it tiny so as to work the very edge of your ligament.
You will get your voice back.
God bless,
Ken McDonald

June 20, 2013
Dear Ken,
I cannot thank-you enough. I just read your email and will begin today. You have explained the exercises very well. My voice is so breathy and still very weak....soft and whispery most of the time. I truly believe your timing with your email is a gift from God and in his perfect timing. I was beginning again to feel so frustrated and praying that possibly another door would open. Thank-you!! Is it ok if I email with questions if I have them concerning this exercise?
Sincerely,
Windy

June 20, 2013
Dear Windy,
Sure on the questions, I would be glad to help. After your first week email me and I will send you your second work out.
God bless,
Ken

Good Vibrations

June 20, 2013
Windy wrote:
Thank-you! I will email you in a week and start the exercises today! I wanted to let you know that I have corresponded with _____ a bit (I do not have her last name in front of me!)...in Philippines as well......I am wondering if you helped her as well. I thought that I recalled her speaking of you!

June 24, 2013
Windy,
I was thinking about the vocal exercise I gave you. I'm not sure of your range so when I said 30-40 minutes that may have been a bit too much. If you can only do 20 minutes it would be OK. If you can go 30-40 good. I just thought I would mention this.
Thanks,
Ken McDonald

June 25, 2013,
Dear Ken,
    Thank-you for your email. Yes, I was actually going to email you yesterday with that very same question! It is very hard for me to sustain 30-40 minutes. I am doing about ten minutes three times a day....is this OK? I also find it hard to not become breathy with voice breaks especially when I am going down the scale with humming.....I find it more difficult going down the scale. I am trying

to be clear and tiny.

Thank-you, Windy

(It is here where I wrote the chapter "For The Very Weak Voice" and emailed it to this student. So as to not repeat it again you may go back to that chapter and read it.)

June 25, 2013
Hi Ken,

Yes, it is hard not hearing my voice for you. When I speak low I seem to have more voice...it is just that I cannot sustain it beyond a few words without going into a whisper and a very breathy voice. Maybe this is why starting low on the keyboard is easier and going up rather than starting high....and going down...this has been hard this week but I will get there...now with your help!! Connie Pike told me that with ABSD...a low pitch was better for recovery so I have tried practicing vocabulary in a low pitch for the last two years or so. My voice before SD was always at a higher pitch and I taught preschool and kindergarten so the higher pitch was always very comfortable for me with the children!! The information that you wrote will be so helpful as I practice these exercises. I will practice the extoning each day and then email you with my progress and questions as to what to do next. I realize from what you have expressed that it will take some time before I begin to notice some improvement! I cannot thank-you enough for all of your help. 1 hope to help others in some way someday with all that I have learned on this journey with SD. It sounds like these exercises that you have given to me have already helped so many with SD! Your book will be a gift to so many that are still trying to recover from SD. I am so grateful for your responses!

I will keep you updated!
Sincerely, Windy

June 25, 2013
Windy,
One thing and I will wait for your response.

This is not in any way critical of Connie Pike it is just an explanation of what she is doing, and for many it has worked. I am not being critical.

You used your voice at a high pitch. That part of your ligament gave out and quit working. So Connie told you to change your pitch and go lower. Why? To find a new place on your ligament that wasn't worn out. Sometimes it works, but it does not correct what was damaged.

The Smolover method takes time because it corrects and strengthens your entire ligament. That part of your ligament that has given out will need to be strengthened and brought back in. This will take time but it corrects the problem, and it does work.

Ken

A Glimpse of The Path

June 26, 2013
Hi Ken,

I would agree with this! For many this works but it does not correct the entire ligament. For me, the method of practicing vocabulary and words in a low pitch just has not corrected the problem over time. The way that you have explained how the ligament becomes damaged (one way or another) and how to strengthen it makes such sense.

I will be in touch soon!
Windy

July 2, 2013
Windy,

I hope you are doing well with your exercises. I have finished my book entitled, "I Can Talk Again." It is being proof read, yet still a ways to go on it.

I was thinking about your voice being breathy when working your voice and thought I would mention this. Your ligament is weak, so when the air is pushed up the ligament blows apart AKA abducts. When you are working your voice and you get to places where it is breathy, back way off on the air and try to make sound with almost no air. It may seem like it is no air. But you want to back off and try to just make sound with very little if any breath. You will be working the very

Good Vibrations

edge of a very weak ligament, but it is the place to start where your ligament can start to strengthen. It will take concentration as you delicately make sound. Listen for the tiny sound and sustain extone for as long as you can. At first it may only be one or two counts. You will work up from there.

For your new exercise sustain extones for 12 counts or as long as you can up to 12 counts. Long sustains build strength and as you ascend you are stretching. So now you will go from stretching only to stretching and building strength.

I was wondering how high are you able to go? What is your highest note? The reason I ask is that if you talked in a high pitch and that part of your ligament is weak, can you get above there and make sound way up high? Maybe you already are doing this, but if not, give it a try. Why? Up high sound is made ligament only. It also aligns the ligament. As you make sound up high, then you will bring it down little by little. The proper working of the ligament will be brought down little by little, and as you do, your voice will come in.

God Bless,
Ken McDonald

A Glimpse of The Path

July 3,, 2013,
Dear Ken,

Thank-you for your email! I actually was going to email you today and let you know that my exercises are going well....daily. I am finding it hard though to sustain the extone for even five counts. I am able to on some notes but then on others....as you described, I become very breathy and my voice begins to break. I can do about eight or so notes as of now, still breathy so I will try what you have described! Should I just continue with the five counts...I thought that on the notes that are more clear with tiny sound I could try and do the longer counts? I am taking a big breath and slowly exhaling with closed lips (my stomach moving inward as I exhale) and extoning with humming sound. Did you find that it took some time with the counts to work up to longer extoning? I am trying to achieve a higher pitch each time....my highest right now is about a middle D or so...I am using a key board (small). I can do about two octaves in highness of notes before I am just using only air. I am so appreciate of all of your feedback with my practice...it really helps!! Everything that you have described makes such sense to me with how it is the ligament that needs to be strengthened with SD. I will continue until I hear back with the five counts!!

Thank-you so much!!
Windy

Good Vibrations

July 3, 2013
Windy,
On the notes you are able sustain extone as long as you can up to 12 counts. On breathy notes do your best. Back off of air and try to make sound with very little breath. On your good notes try some intones for five counts if possible.

Intones can only be made with ligament. Muscle cannot help on intones, so they are excellent in making the ligament work on its own. Intones are very good for SD. You may choke some. That is normal.

Sounds like you are doing well.
Sincerely, Ken

July 4, 2013
Windy wrote:
Hi Ken,
I do have a question concerning intones. How are they done? Do I take a breath inward...sort of like holding my breath? I am not quite sure how to do these exercises and I wanted to ask you before I tried.

Thank-you, Windy

July 4, 2013
Windy,
They are just the opposite of extones. Take a deep breath, then empty your lungs and try to

hum inward. Sometimes you can take a little air in and then start to hum. There really is no wrong way to do it. On intones just make sound anyway you can, then as you get used to it you will be able to sustain intones longer as your ligament strengthens.
Sincerely,
Ken McDonald

July 4, 2013
Thank-you Ken! It sounds like the key is to empty your lungs first and then begin to hum! With the extones, I am humming while I empty my lungs after taking a deep breath. Thank-you! I will begin these tomorrow and I will let you know how they are going with the extone exercises as well.
(The following email from this student I parsed as a reply so it will appear different than the others.)

July 15, 2013
Windy,
(Student)
I thought that I would check in with you this week to let you know that I am still practicing extones and some intones. I am finding the intones a bit more difficult!
(Reply)
Intones are more difficult at first, even for people with normal voice, but they are very good

and essential for your recovery. Intones cannot utilize muscle therefore the ligament must work on its own. There is no wrong way to do intones. Make sound any way you can, and it may only be a short amount of sound. That is a start. The intones will "wake up" your ligament. It does take time.

(Student)

I seem to have more sound when I can extone because of having some breath to carry the sound I believe! I am counting...not quite up to twelve though yet!!

(Reply)

Glad to hear your length of sustain is improving, this is good! Remember to use as little breath as possible, sometimes even seeming like no breath. When the ligament is strong breath can be held back just by the ligament. With a weak ligament you must hold breath back by your lungs not letting much breath out. By the way, you will find in time your lungs will be functioning better. Just a side effect of the work outs.

(Student)

Did you find that it took some time to work up to that count? I will hang in there!!!

(Reply)

Yes, it took time for me, and at the beginning some notes were much better than others. Parts of my ligament were in better shape than other parts. Little by little it will all become equal. Keep

A Glimpse of The Path

trying to go higher. You mentioned that you have a short keyboard. If possible get a full sized keyboard. The visualization of where you are and where you have come from is profitable, as well as your goal.

(Student)

I also find with the intones that it feels like I am pushing more trying to make sound, is this OK?

(Reply)

Yes, on intones make sound any way you can. You are working the flex and as well as the ligament on its own. Air will probably just pass right in with very little sound. You must start somewhere. You are waking up your ligament.

(Student)

I am reading your notes again and again....they are very helpful!!!

(Reply)

One more note. In time your voice may sound and feel weaker. This is normal. Do not panic!

Originally, as your voice weakened you called on helps to prop it up so it would make sound. This is called extrinsic tension, or helps from outside of your larynx. These exercises are designed to work your ligament which is the very heart or center of your voice i.e. larynx. As it begins to strengthen these crutches or props one by one get kicked out, which is good and needed for your ligament to be freed up. When these props go your voice has to stand on its own. When this happens

Good Vibrations

your voice is a bit shaky or weak. Then it will come in, and each time it will be a little stronger and clearer. This cycle will happen many times as your voice strengthens.

Glissando - a sliding of your voice.

When you do a glissando you will slide your voice up and down without stopping. Think of it as making a circle. For the mini glissando you will slide it three times and hold for five counts on your starting note. This is working the very edge of your ligament and smoothing it out so to speak.

A. has had great success with this exercise. Sliding your voice one note up and one note back down, then up and back down. This is done with extones. To begin with, start on your lowest good note. The note that you can make decent sound with. Tiny, Tiny, hold breath back with your lungs, slide your voice up one note. Strike to low key then the next key up, then the original lower key. Slide up, down, up, down and hold five counts. Do not stop on the up or down note. Try to keep your voice sliding up and down, working the very edge of your ligament. As you ascend the keyboard start with the low note and finish on the low note. As you descend from the top, start with the high note and finish with the high note. Speed should be one to two counts on each note, though not stopping on each note. Think of a circle.

Your work out:

A Glimpse of The Path

1. Extone sustains for 12 counts bottom to top and top to bottom. Try to go two notes higher and two notes lower. Hold breath back with lungs.

2. Intones up to 12 counts bottom to top and top to bottom. Make sound as best as you can. Try two notes higher on these as well. Two notes lower not as important.

3. Extone mini glissando - 2 circles, and hold the last for 3 counts if you can. Total of about 9 counts. Ascend and descend the keyboard.

4. Intone sustains 7 counts again - Ascend and descend the keyboard.

5. Extones, 7 counts, up +2 and down +2 - Always finish your workout descending going from top to bottom. You are to bring the ligament down.

Do you find that your neck is sore after a work out?

Sincerely, Ken McDonald

July 16, 2013,
Hi Ken,
Thank-you!! Yes, my neck and shoulders do feel the work out each time!! I have always felt the strain in my upper back as well....I think from trying to push out my voice which I have learned is not good for you!! Over the last few years I have made an effort not to strain and push my voice out....that is why I was left to a whisper most of the time!! I also feel as though I am holding back air in my throat. I have been placing my hand as

well on my abdomen with the intones to make sure I am not letting air out!! My abdomen does still move inward slightly with air (exhaling) when I am practicing the intones but I am working on it!!! I am not too worried because you have said there is really no wrong way to do them as long as I am making sound. I am remembering that each time I practice!!

I practiced the glissando exercise this morning! I was only able to do a few notes but I will get there! I just could not sustain much sound without a break...crack... in my voice moving from note to note!! I held each note counting (for as long as I could) on the top and bottom as you noted. I will practice all that you outlined this week!! I may be emailing you this week if I think of more questions!! I know it will take practice and time.....with your help!!!

Thank-you so much!!
Sincerely,
Windy

August 1, 2013
Hi Ken,

Thank-you for checking!! I have been out of town for the past week or so and I have to say...I was a bit off track with practice while gone! I began yesterday diligently again....I did practice while gone but it was not quite as much!! I am finding that I am able to carry the humm....longer and finding that the gliding is becoming easier up and down with the notes! My voice is still breathy and weak but I am beginning to see some stronger moments of vocalizing!!! Do you believe that it will take a few more months before I see a lot of improvement? I am so thankful as well for all of your prayer along with your guidance.....It means so much to me!

Hope the email goes through!!!

Thank-you!!

Windy

August 1, 2013

Windy,

Yes, I received your email so I know it is working, thank you. I am thrilled to hear you are starting to sense some new vocalizing.

Remember, there may be, and most likely will be, a time where your voice actually gets worse. Do not fear! You will go through these episodes. What is happening when this takes place is that the extrinsic tension, or outside helps you used to try to talk with are dying out. But when they do your ligament has to stand a little more on it's own. Being weak it will be a bit breathy and then come in stronger.

I am glad to hear of your work out fatigue from your shoulders up. It was the same with me. A. told me that was all the extrinsic tension I was using to try to talk. As your ligament strengthens the fatigue will become less and less. Remember though it is going to take time. When I first started, A. told me it would take five years to be completely restored and normal. Looking back she was correct. The exciting part is that you are starting to see improvement. It is bound to happen for you are working your ligament and little by little it will strengthen, align and flex. You are actually restoring and working your voice from the inside out. Your ligament is the very heart of your voice. This is why you work tiny. You are seeking to work your ligament only (modality 1), without help from the vocalis (modality 2) or thyroarytenoid (modality 3)muscles.

Keep doing your workout for a couple more weeks and then I will make some changes to it. In a couple weeks let me know your highest note you can reach on your extones and intones. C4 is middle "C" so C5 is an octave higher etc.

One other thing. As you work your voice, in time you will hear tiny new sounds. They will be clear as well. When you work and hear them go towards the tiny new sound. At first you may not be able to "grab it." Keep trying and then bring it in. That is the new behavior of your ligament and the progress you are wanting. I may be too early in mentioning this to you, but be aware of it. Most of the new sound will be up high. You

will bring it in, and then bring it down note by note. This takes time, as in weeks and months, but it will happen and is a good thing.
God bless,
Ken

September 11, 2013
Hi Ken,
I have been practicing the exercises....one thing that I am still finding is that sometimes I need to breathe before I can go on to the next note.....is that OK? I usually find this when I am trying to glide up and down with the notes...glissando. I know that you told me that even my breathing will improve over time!! I am up as far as about middle C on the keyboard with making humming sounds!! I still have breaks and breathiness but my humming seems to be more clear when practicing...hopefully that is a good sign! Thank-you for checking in with me....I was going to write you too so I am glad that you did!!!
Sincerely,
Windy

September 25, 2013
Windy,

In much of my descriptions of the exercises I have described the form and how to do the exercises which is important. But I am going to

Good Vibrations

recommend something different for you.

First of all, on the glissando just do the whole exercise on one breath and let it be what it is. If your voice cuts out or pops let it and go until you have no breath or if you have enough for the complete exercise.

Secondly, and this one will be hard to do. You need to attempt to make sound any way you can up to two octaves above middle C. You need to "wake your ligament up." When you are doing your work out, somewhere in the middle of it you should try to go two octaves above middle "C" and hum tiny for five counts. Intone or extone it doesn't matter, and you can experiment on each note as you go, but the goal is to make sound for two octaves above middle C. Take it up, no need to bring it down. Then, after a month or so, as you are able do this with intones only. It will take some time, but you need to set this as a goal. It is going to take much work. As your ligament responds then all of your exercises will be done up to this new level.

If you want, start out and go just one octave above middle C. Do this for two or three weeks, and then take it up to two octaves.

Your ligament needs to wake up and begin to function up high because up high is where it can only function on its own. At about one octave above middle C your ligament begins to operate on its own. Do not worry about form. Concentrate and listen for sound on each note. Remember the goal is to have five octaves of sound on intones and extones. This takes years, and though I have sound for five octaves now, yet it is not equal. At the beginning I only had seven or eight notes that I could barely make any sound at all.

I am glad to hear you have some notes that you can hold for 12 counts. You have a good foundation to build on.

    God bless,
    Ken McDonald

September 25, 2013
Hi Ken,
    Thank-you so much! I will do what you have outlined and see if I can go up one to two octaves above middle C. Ken, I have a question that I have been meaning to ask and I finally wrote it down on a sticky note beside my desk so I would not forget!! I am curious to what your thoughts are. When I attended Connie Pikes clinic (both for a private session weekend and for the five day) I met a few people that were told from speech pathologists that when you hum...you should always feel it in your mask area but more importantly...in your mouth. You should feel the

Good Vibrations

hum in your lips when making sound. Connie seemed to feel as well that this was necessary to try and do! I was concerned when practicing because I do not always feel the sound in my lips. I try to bring it to my mask area though in my face. Do you feel that this is necessary with these exercises?

Thank-you for checking in with me and tweaking as we go....it helps more than I can say knowing that you are guiding me with all of this!!!

Sincerely,
Windy

September 25, 2013
Windy,

There were many times when I would go into A.'s studio with me analyzing my voice, my sound, etc. A.'s reply was always, "It is what it is, just do the exercises." She would then say, "The problem is a week ligament." So it is more important to do the exercises than how you do them. You will not hurt your voice. Remember that, you will not hurt your voice. A speech pathologist must focus on form or sound because they do not know how to deal with the ligament itself. But if you get the ligament working correctly then you can concentrate on form and sound. Right now for you it is most important to just do the exercises and attempt when possible to do them tiny.

A Glimpse of The Path

I don't think you can tell at this point, but there is a difference between softly and tiny, so just do the exercises and try not to analyze too much. Listen for the sound when you work your voice, and as new sounds come in go towards the new sounds. I am probably way ahead of that happening with your voice right now, but it will happen. You will not hurt your voice.

If someone is paralyzed it is more important for them to walk, than how they walk. The form comes later. The early stages though are very hard work. I hope this helps.

Ken

October 7, 2013
Hi Ken,

I just have another question if you have time to answer it!! You have been so kind with all of this continued journey to help me succeed with overcoming SD!! I find that it feels like I am holding my breath when practicing...is that OK!! Is that how you felt early on...with ABSD...because of the lack of breath support?

Thank-you!
Windy

Good Vibrations

October 8, 2013
Windy,

   Yes, you have to hold your breath when doing your exercises. Your ligament does not have the strength to stay approximated thus slowing the outflow of breath. You have to hold your breath back in order to keep the sound tiny. As a side note, it is very good exercise for your lungs.

Are you finding any new sounds or any slight improvement in your voice? I am sure you have a long way to go, but is there anything new with your voice, or has anyone said anything to you? I am just curious.   It is important for you to attempt to go two octaves higher above middle C. It is necessary in order for your ligament to align. It aligns up high and then little by little you will bring that new behavior of alignment down.
   I think there may be a possibility that you can get above, on your ligament, where you used to speak, and above that to where your ligament may be functional. This would be up around the two octaves above middle C. Make sound any way you can, there will be no wrong way, and go as high as you can.   It will be hard work, but is necessary. Once you can make sound then you will concentrate on making all the sounds by intone with a sustained of 5 counts to start and work up to 12 counts over time. This will build

strength and alignment, both of which are needed at this point. Attempt this at the middle or end of your workout.

God bless,
Ken

October 9, 2013
Hi Ken,

Thank-you for clarifying with my breath. It just feels like I am struggling to hold my breath....it is hard work!! At times Ken, I am noticing that if I am speaking....my sounds are stronger with my voice. I am able to sustain a conversation somewhat longer than just a few words. I still cannot project that much and my voice is weak and breathy but I am noticing (my husband as well!!) that once in awhile my voice appears to be holding more sounds...more strongly than a few months ago!! Hopefully, this is a good sign!!

I am practicing daily....trying to go above middle C......two octaves. Sometimes nothing comes out when I attempt but I am still going higher!! I am holding for about seven counts on some notes now!! I will continue to keep you updated on my progress!

I know it will be a slow process!! It will be worth the effort....I believe this!!

Blessings to you as well!!
Thank-you,
Windy

Good Vibrations

This student, as you can see, I have been working with for just a few months at the date of this writing 10/7/2013. I included it because it is more detailed in the correspondence and illustrates the fears and questions that come up as a person begins to work their voice.

A DIFFERENT STUDENT WHOM I NAMED "BREEZY"

I am now going to list another students' emails. This student responded extremely quickly to the work out.

This is about seven months after starting to work the voice:

April 5, 2012,
Breezy wrote:
Hi Ptr. McDonald,
Thank you so much! It's reassuring to know that you went through the same phase and it means that i'm on the right track :-)
For my daily voice exercise, I do:
Approx. 1 hour (total):
5 mins = 1st warm up: Extone for 2 seconds, Intone for 2 seconds. From G (2 Gs below Middle C) to D (2 Ds above Middle C). I do about 3 rounds of this.
5 mins = 2nd warm up: Fifths. Extone from G (2

A Glimpse of The Path

Gs below Middle C) & 5th note. And then I reach until A (1st A above Middle C) & 5th note. I do this about 3 rounds.

25 mins = EXTONE for 15 secs, from G (2 Gs below Middle C) to F (2 Fs above Middle C). Then start from there and go down again. I think I do about 5 rounds.

25 mins = INTONE for 5 secs, from G (2 Gs below Middle C) to D (2 Ds above Middle C). Start from there and go down to where I started. 5 rounds also.

5 mins = Cool down: I start from D (2 Ds above Middle C). Extone 2 secs, Intone 2 secs, Extone 2 secs. Intone 2 secs, Extone 2 secs, Intone 2 secs. 2 rounds.

I've noticed in my cool down that my voice seems to "lock" when I do the extone. It's like it got used to doing the Intones then when I do the Extone in between, it locks and does not produce sound. But after a while of continuing the exercise, the voice comes out.

I hope I'm doing it as closely to your regimen as possible

Date: Wednesday, April 11, 2012,
Breezy,
On the warm up - Extone 2 seconds and intone 2 seconds, but do this twice making a total of four and then one more extone and hold for five counts. (Remember Tiny when possible) You only

Good Vibrations

need to do this once for a warm up but continue to try for two notes higher and lower. Try for the G 2 octaves above middle C. Eventually you will try for three octaves above middle C and two octaves below middle C making a total of five octaves. Keep stretching.

On the fifths - alternate the fifths intone and then extone all the way up. Do a fifth intone and then the next note up do it extone alternating all the way up. You only need to do this once a work out. Remember to slide your voice on this workout, that is very important. Think of moving it in a circle up around and down and around back up. On the fifths, work your voice alternating each note going up, and then do it also down to as low as possible. Once up and once down.

The rest of the work out looks good. I know it is hard but try to do your intones as long as possible, up to 15 seconds. If some notes are longer than others go ahead and hold it on those notes and work the others as long as you are able.

God bless,
Bro. Ken

Apr 11, 2012, (6th month of therapy)
Breezy wrote:
Hi Ptr. McDonald,

Thank you very much for these new voice exercises! I will do them. My voice was better 2 days ago until yesterday. Today, it was a bit bad. But now I am confident that the voice up and down is a cycle :-)

I will continue to keep you posted.

Warm regards,

Breezy

Hi Ptr. McDonald,

How are you? :p I'm still doing the vocal exercises 1 Hour everyday, 6 days a week. My voice continues to improve. And yes there are cycles of "good voice-bad voice", which is quite normal.

Thanks so much for your guidance. I'm starting to really feel that I'm truly on my way to recovery; however slow or time-consuming it may be. But I'm so very grateful that God has guided me to meet you.

I can now do about an 6-10 seconds of intone, depending on the note. You are right, some notes I can do for 6 seconds, others I can do 10. I just try to do the maximum of each intone. I experience less "locking of the voice" now when I'm doing my alternate Intone-Extone at the end of the therapy.

Last May 25th, I realized I've been doing the exercises for 6 mos now. I started Nov. 25. All the effort for the past months are paying off!

How about you? How are you doing?
Warm regards,
Breezy

On Jul 11, 2012, (7th Month of therapy)
Dear Ptr. McDonald,
Hello! I'm on my 7th month of voice therapy with you. I'm still doing the same voice therapy program from your last April email. I've increased the notes 2 notes up and 2 notes down. The lowest I've reached now is 2 C's below middle C. And the highest is now 2 F's above middle C.

For the Extone, majority of the notes I can do 12-15 seconds, some especially the lowest notes I could only do about 7-8 seconds. I still couldn't reach the 15 seconds for Intone, so I'm still working on it. It varies per note, but I do an average of 5 seconds to 10 seconds in the Intone. And mostly it is about me running out of breath, not about the vocal cords giving in. I can feel my cords getting stronger. So far, my voice has been pretty good. :-) I still have bad voice days, but not as bad as before.

How about you? How are you doing? Hope all is well. Thank you so much for pointing me to the right way..
Warm regards,
Breezy

A Glimpse of The Path

Thursday, July 12, 2012
Dear Breezy,
I had the opportunity to go to my voice teacher today and it went very well, She reminded me of some things which I will pass on to you.

Remember to do tiny and clear. You are trying to work the edge of the ligament only, so tiny and clear on the sound. Clear sound will be hard down low so just do your best and if the air flows through let it. Try to stay away from hard heavy sounds especially down low.

Also, you can back off to 7 seconds on all exercises. It is not needed to work for a complete hour. Half hour will do, but if you go an hour it is OK. I have a tendency to work too hard, and she reminded me of that.

Here is a new exercise. Start low as you can and hum lightly outward moving up one note then down one note, back up one and down again, then back up and hold for three seconds. Move your way up the keyboard to as high as you can and then do the same things downward. You hum a note then slide up one note and down humming the whole time. This is done three times and then held for three seconds on the down side, starting note. Then start at the next note higher. Remember to do tiny and clear.

Remember it takes time. You are doing well. It took me two years of time with an expert teacher

to progress and then another year to be fairly normal. Don't quit.
God bless,
Bro. Ken
Jn 9:4

Date: Friday, July 13, 2012,
Dear Ptr. McDonald,
I checked again and the lowest I could do was only 1 C below middle C, and the highest is 2 Bs above middle C... I remember the placement of the keys in the keyboard, but don't remember much the names of the keys.. Haha.
I am doing your reminder – tiny and clear. It is helping! I do have the tendency to force the sound out. Thanks for the tip! I also tried the new exercise. I'll keep you posted!
Warm regards,
Breezy

Wednesday, August 29, 2012 (9th Month therapy)
Dear Ptr. McDonald,
Hello! I wasn't able to do my voice therapy for about a week (or 10 days) because I went out of town with friends doing backpacking! :-) Birthday treat for myself. I did some humming while I was gone, though.
Now I've started the voice therapy again, been doing it for about 4 days now. My voice is doing

well yesterday and today. The previous week it hasn't been well. Especially after drinking coffee. My dad bought this new kind of coffee and it tasted good so I drank every morning during breakfast. I did it for 3-4 days straight. And I noticed my voice got weak! I'm not sure if it has a relation to it, but I have a feeling it does! Because I drank wheatgrass and my voice started coming back again. Coffee might be too acidic? Have you encountered something like this before?
:-0

Hope you're good! Just like me, I'm generally doing better these past months. I still can't do regular work, though. Good thing I have a shop. God is good to me! He led me to people like you who guided me.

Warm regards,
Breezy

On Nov. 25, 2012,
Hi Ptr. McDonald,

Yesterday, November 25th was my 1st year of the voice exercises!

I actually stopped doing my exercises for about 1.5-2 months, because I've been traveling a lot and I became lazy! Big mistake! My voice was holding up very well so I didn't bother (again, my bad) and it held up for about 2 months! Now I felt my voice begin to quiver.. I'm back to my exercises!

But at least when my voice turned bad again, I'm somehow at peace because I know I just need to do my exercises again faithfully. And give it time to solidify the strong voice. At least I know the way how to get better. Thanks so much for leading and guiding me and for showing me the way!!

Hope you are doing good as well.

I'm about to get married in January next year! And I've been busy with the preparations! But I'll make time for my vocal exercises. :-)

Warm regards,
Breezy

Saturday, December 8, 2012
(Nov. 25 – One Year of therapy!)

Dear Breezy,
Sorry for the delay in getting back to you.

It is good to know the exercises work and you don't have to live in fear. Remember to do them tiny to work the very edge of your ligament. Tiny clear sound. When ligament is weak it may take more than tiny but as it strengthens bring it down to tiny.

There is one more exercise I can give you which is this:

As low as you can, after your warm ups, start with tiny sound slide up only one note, and slide down one note and back up one note and then back down one note, go back up one note and back down one note and hold, if you can, for three counts. Do this all the way up to as high as you can go. Then do the same thing down but start on the high note and go one note down and then one note back up three times so you end on the up note. Keep the sound going through the whole exercise if you can.

Slide up down, up down, up down, hold for three. This will consist of humming tiny for nine counts. Then from as high as you can move downward. Do this only once per session.

My instructor told me that this exercise was one of the most effective exercises for Spasmodic Dysphonia. If you need to then cut out one of the other exercises and do this one, but continue with the warm ups first, and the cool downs last.

God bless,
Bro. Ken McDonald

Saturday, December 8, 2012
(Nov. 25 – One Year of therapy!)
Hi Ptr. McDonald,

Thanks so much! I'll remember clear & tiny... :-) I have been receiving some emails from other SD patients who have seen my blog about SD. I've been sharing the things you've taught me. Hope it's OK :-) I've shared about A. V. there also if they'd like to get in touch with her directly.

Good Vibrations

You're really helping a lot of people! And yes, it removes the fear in my heart knowing that there is a slow but sure way to recovery.

Warm regards,
Breezy

March 5, 2013
Dear Ptr. McDonald
Hello! How have you been? :-) I got married this January :-) I've attached our picture! We went to China for our honeymoon, the Great Wall was amazing!

My voice has been generally steady the past 2 months. But still, I find it easier to talk to people I know and am comfortable with. There are times when I need to ask something from the grocery saleswoman that some voice and some air would come out, instead of clear voice. But it's now very much manageable compared to before. When I was at the altar during the wedding, saying my vows, I was so glad I had some voice! :-) It seems odd, but when I talk to someone face to face, I sound better than when I'm given a microphone to talk into.

But in the end, I was able to say my vows and I'm glad! Thank you very much! :-)

When I went abroad and couldn't bring my piano or laptop, what I did was to record the voice exercises in my mobile phone. That's what I played and exercised with! :-)

Hope all is well with you,
Breezy

Good Vibrations

16

Origin Of The Smolover Method AKA Vocal Behavior Training

Here is a description of the origin and background of the Smolover method. This is taken from the book, *Sing Your Best*, by Raymond Smolover.

History of the Smolover Method:

>The Smolover Method of vocal behavior training is the result of over 50 years of research and teaching. Dr. Smolover's musical training began with the study of the violin at age 8 and voice at age 14. He went on to study music education at Carnegie Mellon University. After serving in the Army Air Corps, he moved to New

York to pursue a professional singing career, and to work as a voice-teaching associate of Dr. Douglas Stanley, author of The Science of Voice. He subsequently opened his own teaching studio and began graduate work in voice research at Columbia University. This research involved the study of voice physiology and anatomy, dissection of larynxes with medical students, and observation of laryngologists at work on living voices. Dr. Smolover worked closely with a number of laryngologists (notably, Dr. Wilbur J. Gould), professors of vocal pedagogy (including Dr. Craig Timberlake), speech therapists and other specialists in voice function. He also worked with Dr. R. Douglas Greer, professor of psychology, music and education. During this time he continued teaching singers of all ages and musical styles and observing the effects of training on vocal development.

The Smolover Method is based on the identification of three distinct vocal sounds, observable in Pre-verbal children and attributable to the functioning of three sections of the vocal cords: the vocal ligament, the vocalis muscles and the thyroarytenoid muscle. To underscore the physiological underpinnings of each of the three sound types, Dr. Smolover uses the term "modalities" rather than "registers." In effect, they are three different modes of vibration of the vocal cords and are characterized by identifiably different sound qualities. He observed that, through training, a singer could produce sounds in the three modalities beyond what was usually expected of pitch registers. **His use of intoning in vocal training was inspired by its successful use in speech therapy to treat spasmodic dysphonia,** a vocal disorder characterized by laryngeal spasm preventing normal speech. He found that when extoning produced no cord vibration, intoning reduced tension sufficiently to allow the cords to vibrate, **eventually enabling patients to resume normal speech and singing.** (Emphasis Added) The use of intoning in this vocal training method has been very important in enabling students to bypass extrinsic tension sufficiently to access pitches in the two octaves above C6. Very soft humming in this range has proved to be and exceptionally effective method of isolating and developing the response of the vocal ligament.

With the 1983 publication of his doctoral dissertation, *Vocal Behavior Analysis and Modification Under Conditions of Expiratory and Inspiratory Phonation*, Dr. Smolover was able to demonstrate quantitatively his theory of vocal modalities. He showed that the three modalities could be successfully recognized aurally (Vocal Behavior Analysis), that trained students could measurably improve their pitch range in the intrinsic muscles of the voice—facilitated by intoning—the less tension exhibited in the extrinsic muscles (Expiatory and Inspiratory Phonation). Copies of the study may be obtained by contacting Columbia University Library. During the years of his research, Dr. Smolover was affiliated with the International Association for Research in Singing, founded by John Large, who solicited his dissertation for publication in the Journal of Research in Singing. Dr. Smolover later became the Director of the Foundation for Research in Singing, a sister organization dedicated to encouraging voice research and developing applications to vocal instruction.[17]

It is with fond memories that I think back on the hours of work I spent in my instructor's studio. We prayed together, laughed and cried. She "tortured" me and worked my voice with skill and patience.

When I canceled all my meetings and went into therapy, I was resigned to being homeless and having my wife and daughter living in another state just so they could have a place to stay. These were all fears, but it is what I was mentally prepared for. I have no regrets for leaving it all so I could get my voice back.

In the Bible it says, "God turned the curse into a blessing unto thee." It is my prayer that my curse of having SD can now be turned into a blessing to you. May the Lord bless you as you work to regain your voice.

Good Vibrations

17

The Most Important Step

In order to get your voice back your are going to need some help, and that help must come from the One who created you. This chapter is about taking the first step in getting His help.

Dear friend, would you let me ask you one of the most important questions that you will ever be asked in this life? The question is this, *"Do you know that you are going to Heaven when you die?"*

Perhaps you say that no one knows where they are going when they die. Well, St. Peter knew that he was going to Heaven for he said that he was born again, **"kept by the power of God,"** and that he had an incorruptible inheritance reserved in Heaven. St. John knew that he was going to Heaven for he said, **"Now are we the sons of**

Good Vibrations

God...and we know that we shall be like Him." "These things have I written unto you that believe on the name of the Son of God; that ye may know that ye have eternal life..." (1John 5:13)

Not only did St. Peter and St. John know where they were going when they died, but St. Paul also knew for he said that he had a **"desire to depart, and to be with Christ; which is far better."** And of course Jesus Christ said, **"I go unto my Father."**

All of these men, as well as the Son of God, knew where they were going when they died. If they knew, you can know also. In the Bible St. John wrote again, **"These things have I written unto you that believe on the name of the Son of God; that ye may know that ye have eternal life..."** (1 Jn 5:13)

Do you know that you have eternal life? Do you know that you are going to Heaven when you die?

Let me start at the very beginning. The person you are going to have to deal with is called, "the Word," and He is the Creator of all things.

> John 1:1 In the beginning was the Word, and the Word was with God, and the Word was God.
>
> 2 The same was in the beginning with God.
>
> 3 All things were made by him; and without him was not any thing made

that was made. 4 In him was life; and the life was the light of men.

He is also righteous. In Heaven they worship Him.

> Rev. 4:8 And the four beasts had each of them six wings about him; and they were full of eyes within: and they rest not day and night, saying, Holy, holy, holy, Lord God Almighty, which was, and is, and is to come.

His name is the Son of God, the Lord Jesus Christ.

> "But unto the Son he saith, Thy throne, O God, is for ever and ever: a sceptre of righteousness is the sceptre of thy kingdom." (Heb. 1:8)

The Lord Jesus Christ is Holy. That means He has never sinned one time. There is no spot nor blemish in the Lord Jesus Christ. He is absolutely perfect. Along with that, Heaven is also perfect. It is a place of joy, happiness, light, and righteousness. In Heaven:

> Rev. 21:4 And God shall wipe away all tears from their eyes; and there shall be no more death, neither sorrow, nor crying, neither shall there be any more pain: for the

> former things are passed away.
> 5 And he that sat upon the throne said, Behold, I make all things new. And he said unto me, Write: for these words are true and faithful.

This is just a glimpse of Heaven but it gives a glimpse of a place where it can honestly be written as an epitaph, *"...and they lived happily ever after."* Doesn't that sound like a place you would like to spend eternity in?

Heaven is beautiful because the God of Heaven is holy, the place called Heaven is holy, and the people of Heaven are holy. My desire in writing this is to tell you how you can know when you die you will make it to this beautiful place called Heaven. Then it can be written of you, he or she lived happily ever after.

This brings us to the subject of holiness. Are you holy? Are you righteous? Are you a good person? To answer the first two questions I would think it would be easy to answer, *"No."* You are not holy, and you are not righteous. But maybe your answer to the third question is, *"Yes."* You might say that you are a good person. You're nice to others and try to help folks when you can. That is a good thing.

When it comes to holiness though, how do we judge what is holy? How do we know what holiness is? To answer these two questions we

The Most Important Step

must go back in time about 3500 years to a mountain in Arabia. It is a mountain called Mt. Sinai. On that mountain is a man called Moses. The Lord God has called him there, and camped below in the plain is a nation God has called out of Egypt named Israel.

The top of that mountain can be seen today in 2017. It is in Arabia and has been burnt black, and is a reminder of the event that I am about to tell you of.

Moses went up onto the mount, and God came down in fire on the top of that mount and gave Moses the Ten Commandments. These Ten Commandments are a glimpse of holiness, or should I say, the standard by which holiness is judged. I am going to use only four of the ten and let's see how you measure up to holiness.

> **1. Ex. 20:7 Thou shalt not take the name of the LORD thy God in vain; for the LORD will not hold him guiltless that taketh his name in vain.**

This is the third commandment. To take the Lord's name in vain is called blasphemy and it is very serious. Have you ever taken the Lord's name in vain? In other words have you ever said, *"Oh my God,"* or *"Jesus Christ,"* or *"Lord God Almighty,"* or just *"Jesus?"*

Good Vibrations

Have you ever said any of these in vain, or other variations? How many times in your life have you taken His name in vain? In vain would mean that you just said His name without using it in a sentence, thus in vain. Since this is called blasphemy, then you would be called a blasphemer.

If you have broken this commandment then you are a blasphemer.

2. Ex. 20:15 Thou shalt not steal.

This is the eighth commandment. Have you ever stolen anything in your life? Stop and think about this. Have you ever, without permission, downloaded any music, or anything that was copyrighted? Have you ever taken something that was not yours? Size does not matter. From a piece of candy to millions of dollars, have you ever stolen something?

It doesn't matter what religion you are, for these laws are written on your heart. You know instinctively that it is wrong to take something that is not yours.

What does God call someone who steals? They are called a thief. So then if you have stolen anything you are a thief. You are guilty of breaking God's law when He wrote, **"Thou shalt not steal."**

If you have broken both of these

commandments, then you are a blasphemer and a thief. Keep in mind this is only two of the ten commandments.

3. Ex. 20:14 Thou shalt not commit adultery.

This is to have sex with someone who is not your spouse, thus it is to have sex outside of marriage.

Jesus, who was God manifest in the flesh, went even farther and stated, Matt. 5:28 **"But I say unto you, That whosoever looketh on a woman to lust after her hath committed adultery with her already in his heart."**

Adultery is now committed in your heart by looking on someone and lusting after them sexually, as well as the physical act of fornicating with someone. Fornication is what it is called when sex is committed outside of marriage. This would include Sodomy. Have you ever done that?

If you have, even if just once, then you are an adulterer, or could also be called a fornicator. If you have broken all three of these commandments then you are a blasphemer, thief and a fornicator.

4. Matt. 19:18 "...Thou shalt not bear false witness."

Also known as, **"Thou shalt not lie."**

Have you ever told a lie? To speak a false

Good Vibrations

witness is to tell a lie. A witness tells what he or she knows. To be a false witness is to not speak or tell the truth about what you know. Have you ever done that? How many times have you done that in your life? 1 time? 10? 100? 1000? Etc.?

A person who tells lies, is called a liar. Then you are a liar.

If you have transgressed all four of these commandments then you are a blasphemer, a thief, a fornicator and a liar. Do you think God will allow you into Heaven? What kind of place would Heaven be if God allowed blasphemers, thieves, fornicators and liars into it? I'll tell you, it wouldn't be a holy place, and it wouldn't be Heaven.

With just four out of ten commandments, we have had a glimpse of holiness. The Bible states, **"Wherefore the law is holy, and the commandment holy, and just, and good." Rom. 7:12 "...but I am carnal, sold under sin." Rom. 7:14**

The truth of the matter is that you are not holy, nor are you even good, and neither am I. We all are sinners and have broken God's commandments.

The Bible says,

> 1Cor. 6:9 Know ye not that the unrighteous shall not inherit the kingdom of God? Be not deceived:

The Most Important Step

neither fornicators, nor idolaters, nor adulterers, nor effeminate, nor abusers of themselves with mankind,

10 Nor thieves, nor covetous, nor drunkards, nor revilers, nor extortioners, shall inherit the kingdom of God.

Rev. 21:8 But the fearful, and unbelieving, and the abominable, and murderers, and whoremongers, and sorcerers, and idolaters, and all liars, shall have their part in the lake which burneth with fire and brimstone: which is the second death.

Rev. 20:14 And death and hell were cast into the lake of fire. This is the second death.

15 And whosoever was not found written in the book of life was cast into the lake of fire.

If you die right now, according to the word of God, where will you go? Have you ever told a lie? Then you are a liar and according to the Bible you will go to the lake of fire.

Is that where you want to go when you die? If you are in your right mind then you do not want to end up in the Lake of Fire for all eternity.

Good Vibrations

Is there a way to be saved from going to Hell? If you have been honest with yourself about those four commandments, then you know that you have broken at least one of them. The Bible says, **For whosoever shall keep the whole law, and yet offend in one point, he is guilty of all.** James 2:10 Then according to the word of God you are guilty of breaking God's law and thus unable of your own self to enter Heaven.

In your present condition you will one day stand before your Creator and Judge who will pronounce the judgement, *"Guilty!"* The punishment for you is that you will be cast into Hell and then later cast into the Lake of Fire. That is what you deserve, and that is what I deserve as well, but this is where the good news begins.

Good News

Jesus Christ was God manifest in the flesh. That means Jesus Christ was fully God. He came to this earth being born of the virgin Mary, and became a man. While on this earth He never broke God's law one time. Jesus Christ lived a perfect life according to His law. Jesus Christ is Holy. How do I know this? Because after He was crucified on the cross, our Lord arose from the dead after spending three days and three nights in the heart of the earth.

If Jesus Christ had sinned one time, then He

never would have been able to rise from the dead. He would have been just like you and me. But He did rise from the dead and was seen by over 500 people after He arose from the dead.

Jesus Christ saw you long before you were ever around. He saw you and He loved you.

> **For God so loved the world, that he gave his only begotten Son, that whosoever believeth in him should not perish, but have everlasting life. John 3:16**

God gave his Son; how? He gave him when Jesus died on the cross as the sacrifice for your sins. Jesus Christ took the punishment of your sins upon Himself, and shed His blood as the perfect payment for your sins. The sins that you committed when you transgressed those commandments have all been paid for.

> Rom. 5:6 For when we were yet without strength, in due time Christ died for the ungodly.
>
> 7 For scarcely for a righteous man will one die: yet peradventure for a good man some would even dare to die.
>
> 8 But God commendeth his love toward us, in that, while we were yet

> sinners, Christ died for us.
>
> 9 Much more then, being now justified by his blood, we shall be saved from wrath through him.

While you were a sinner, Jesus Christ loved you and died for you on the cross. He also shed His blood as the payment for your sins, but you must pick up the payment. **"For the wages of sin is death; but the gift of God is eternal life through Jesus Christ our Lord."** (Rom. 6:23)

Wages are given as payment for something that you have worked for. Those commandments that you have broken have earned you death. That is your payment, that is what you have worked for.

A gift is something that you do not work for. A gift is given free of charge after the giver worked to purchase it or to make it. The gift that I am writing about here is eternal life. Do you want to live forever? Do you want to go to Heaven when you die? It is a free gift, but there is one catch. You must receive the Lord Jesus Christ in order to obtain eternal life.

Eternal life is not obtained through baptism, church membership, getting rid of bad karma, or any other works. It is obtained through our Lord Jesus Christ. He is the One that paid the price. You must receive Jesus Christ as your very own personal Saviour.

The Most Important Step

John 1:10 He was in the world, and the world was made by him, and the world knew him not.

11 He came unto his own, and his own received him not.

12 But as many as received him, to them gave he power to become the sons of God, even to them that believe on his name:

13 Which were born, not of blood, nor of the will of the flesh, nor of the will of man, but of God.

So how do you receive Jesus Christ? If you can't see Him, feel Him or touch Him, how can you receive Him? **"For whosoever shall call upon the name of the Lord shall be saved."** (Rom. 10:13)

You must pray and ask Jesus Christ to forgive you of your sins; to wash you from your sins in His own blood; and ask Him to come into your heart and save you from your sins. **"And from Jesus Christ, who is the faithful witness, and the first begotten of the dead, and the prince of the kings of the earth. Unto him that loved us, and washed us from our sins in his own blood."** (Rev. 1:5)

Summary:
1. You have broken God's Holy Commands. Blasphemer, Thief, Fornicator or Liar - Guilty! Headed for the Lake of Fire.

2. Jesus Christ died for your sins, was buried and three days later arose from the grave proving that He was God manifest in the flesh. He paid for all of your sins. Your ticket to Heaven is all paid for, now you must receive Jesus Christ into your heart in order to claim the payment for your sins.

3. You must call upon the Lord Jesus Christ to forgive you of your sins and to wash you in His blood. You must ask the Lord Jesus Christ to come into your heart and save you.

Here is a simple prayer to pray. Remember though, that by faith in what God said, you are talking to Jesus Christ from your heart. Reciting this prayer will not save you. You must realize that you are talking to your Saviour, Jesus Christ. He is the One you need to forgive you and to save you. He promised to save you if you call upon His name and God cannot lie. The best way you know how pray this prayer out loud. Talk to the Lord out loud.

> *Dear Lord Jesus Christ. I come to you as a sinner who has broken your commandments. I am guilty. I believe you died on the cross and paid for my sins. Please forgive me of my sins. Please wash me*

The Most Important Step

> *throughly in your blood. And dear Jesus, please come into my heart and save me. I don't want to go to the Lake of Fire. Thank you for dying for me on the cross and thank you for saving me. In your name, Lord Jesus, I ask these things, Amen.*

If you prayed a prayer like that one and meant it, then according to the word of God you are saved from eternal damnation. I now ask you, "Where are you now going when you die?"

> **Rom. 10:13** For whosoever shall call upon the name of the Lord shall be saved.

> **John 6:37** All that the Father giveth me shall come to me; and him that cometh to me I will in no wise cast out.

These are both prescious promises from the word of God.

Good Vibrations

Bibliography

1. *Bailey's Head & Neck Surgery: Otolaryngology*, Vol. 1, 5th Edition ©2014 Lippincott Williams & Wilkins; Chapter 71, Voice Therapy for the Treatment of Voice Disorders, Jackie Gartner-Schmidt, Pg 1056.

2. Lessac-Madsen Resonant Voice Therapy (LMRVT): A Brief Description and Review Elvadine R. Seligmann Summer Vocology Institute 2005, Denver, CO USA; http://www.ellieseligmann.com/essays/lmrvt.htm (Accessed 8/28/2017).

3. *Sing Your Best*, Smolover & Bertoli, Alfred, 2006, Pg 5.

4. http://www.gbmc.org/vocalwarm-up (accessed 8/28/2017).

5. *Free to Speak II*, Connie M. Pike, Createspace. Kindle Edition Pgs 54-55.

6. *Exercise for the Voice*, Dr. Barbara Mathis, http://www.voiceteacher.com/mathis2.html (accessed 8/28/2017).

7. *Training the Contralto Voice: Developing Diagnostic*

Tools for Understanding a Rare Voice Type, David L Jones, http://www.voiceteacher.com/contralto.html (accessed 8/28/2017).

8. *Sing Your Best*, Smolover & Bertoli, Alfred, 2006, Pg 14.

9. http://www.telegraph.co.uk/news/celebritynews/9725893/Julie-Andrews-famous-singing-voice-ruined-by-throat-operation.html (accessed 8/28/2017).

10. *Career Crises Intervention and the Opera Singer*, David L. Jones, http://www.voiceteacher.com/career_crisis.html (accessed 8/28/2017).

11. *Voice Disorders and their Management*, by Margaret Fawcus, 1986 Croom Helm Ltd., Originally Published by Chapman & Hall in 1991. Pages 278-279.

12. *The Actor Speaks: Voice and the Performer*, Patsy Rodenburg, ©2000 Patsy Rodenburg, St. Martins Press, 175 Fifth Ave., New York, New York 10010, Pg 80.

13. *Parkinson's Disease*, Ronald F. Pfeiffer, Zbigniew K. Wszolek, Manuchair Ebadi December 28, 2004 by CRC Press, Page 813.

14. *Sing Your Best*, Smolover & Bertoli, Alfred, 2006, Pg 12.

15. *Coffin's Sounds of Singing: Principles and Applications of Vocal Techniques with Chromatic Vowel Chart*, Berton Coffin ©1976, 1987, 2002, Scarecrow Press, Inc., Pg 132.

16. *Bailey's Head & Neck Surgery: Otolaryngology*, Vol. 1, 5th Edition ©2014 Lippincott Williams & Wilkins; Chapter 71, Voice Therapy for the Treatment of Voice Disorders, Jackie Gartner-Schmidt, Pg 1051.

17. *Sing Your Best*, Smolover & Bertoli, Alfred, 2006, Pg 46.